Communications
in Computer and Information Science   1387

More information about this series at http://www.springer.com/series/7899

Martina Ziefle · Nick Guldemond ·
Leszek A. Maciaszek (Eds.)

Information and Communication Technologies for Ageing Well and e-Health

6th International Conference, ICT4AWE 2020
Prague, Czech Republic, May 3–5, 2020
Revised Selected Papers

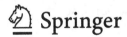 Springer

Editors
Martina Ziefle
RWTH Aachen University
Aachen, Germany

Nick Guldemond
Erasmus University
Rotterdam, The Netherlands

Leszek A. Maciaszek
Institute of Business Informatics
Wrocław University of Economics
Wrocław, Poland

Department of Computing
Macquarie University
Sydney, NSW, Australia

ISSN 1865-0929   ISSN 1865-0937   (electronic)
Communications in Computer and Information Science
ISBN 978-3-030-70806-1   ISBN 978-3-030-70807-8   (eBook)
https://doi.org/10.1007/978-3-030-70807-8

This Springer imprint is published by the registered company Springer Nature Switzerland AG
The registered company address is: Gewerbestrasse 11, 6330 Cham, Switzerland

Preface

The present book includes extended and revised versions of a set of selected papers from the 6th International Conference on Information and Communication Technologies for Ageing Well and e-Health (ICT4AWE 2020), held as a web-based event due to the Covid-19 pandemic, from 3–5 May.

ICT4AWE 2020 received 50 paper submissions from 30 countries, of which 14% were included in this book. The papers were selected by the event chairs and their selection was based on a number of criteria that included the classifications and comments provided by the program committee members, the session chairs' assessment and also the program chairs' global view of all papers included in the technical program. The authors of selected papers were then invited to submit a revised and extended version of their papers having at least 30% innovative material.

The International Conference on Information and Communication Technologies for Ageing Well and e-Health aims to be a meeting point for those that study age- and health-related quality of life and apply information and communication technologies to helping people stay healthier, more independent and active at work or in their community. ICT4AWE facilitates the exchange of information and dissemination of best practices, innovation and technical improvements in the fields of age and health care, education, psychology, social coordination and ambient assisted living. From e-Health to intelligent systems and ICT devices, the conference is a vibrant discussion and collaboration platform for all those that work in research and development and in companies involved in promoting the quality of life and well-being of people, by providing room for research and industrial presentations, demos and project descriptions.

The papers selected to be included in this book contribute to the understanding of relevant trends of current research on Information and Communication Technologies for Ageing Well and e-Health. The contributions can be assigned to three main thematic areas: (1) Ageing well - social and human sciences perspective (2) Ambient intelligence and independent living, and (3) Telemedicine and e-Health.

Within the first category, the social and human sciences perspective on ageing well, Khalid Al-Naime, Akash Gupta and, Adnan Al-Anbuky propose an IoT environment for long-term monitoring of hip fracture rehabilitation-related activity movements and show that the environment can offer flexibility for different movement monitoring, analysis and visualisation applications. In a second paper within this category, another study contributes to the understanding of media use in social relationship management of a group of highly educated and socially connected older adults aged 65+ in Switzerland. The paper (authored by Veronika Hämmerle, Cora Pauli, Rhea Braunwalder and Sabina Misoch) contributes to research that combines established life-span perspectives on ageing with current environmental theories and media usage. A final study in this category, provided by Esther Ruf, Stephanie Lehmann and Sabina Misoch, deals with the usage of robots to support older adults in everyday or care activities and looks at robot acceptance criteria in this regard. The second thematic category, dealing with ambient intelligence and independent living, offers three research papers. Using an explorative user study approach, Esther Ruf and colleagues from the Eastern Switzerland University of Applied Sciences investigate whether a socially assistive robot could be a practical solution to motivate older adults living independently to exercise regularly in order to promote physical health and activity. Another paper, authored by Manola Ricciuti, Gianluca Ciattaglia, Adelmo De Santis, Ennio Gambi and, Linda Senigagliesi from the University of Ancona, Italy, is concerned with the detection of vital parameters, to be used for constant home monitoring for the elderly. It explores the accuracy and validity of contactless methodologies for heart rate monitoring. The aim of the third paper, authored by Christos Goumopoulos and Ioannis Igoumenakis from the University of the Aegean, Greece, is to provide insights on the design and implementation of ontology-based healthcare applications using a game platform for mild cognitive impairment rehabilitation. The last paper, allocated within the third category, telemedicine and e-Health, is provided by Marco Alfano, Davide Taibi, Biagio Lenzitti and Markus Helfert. The research introduces FACILE, a custom search engine that enables both medical experts and non-experts to easily specify medical information requirements in terms of language level, specific information sought and information quality in order to get reliable and required medical information on the Web.

We would like to thank all the authors for their contributions, and also the reviewers, who have helped to ensure the quality of this publication.

May 2020

Martina Ziefle
Nick Guldemond
Leszek Maciaszek

Organization

Conference Chair

Leszek Maciaszek   Wrocław University of Economics, Poland
and Macquarie University, Australia

Program Co-chairs

Nick Guldemond   Erasmus University, The Netherlands
Martina Ziefle   RWTH-Aachen University, Germany

Program Committee

Mehdi Adda	Université du Québec à Rimouski, Canada
Sandra Baldassarri	University of Zaragoza, Spain
Giacinto Barresi	Istituto Italiano di Tecnologia, Italy
Karsten Berns	TU Kaiserslautern, Germany
Laurent Billonnet	ENSIL-ENSCI - Université de Limoges, France
Philipp Brauner	RWTH Aachen University, Germany
Jane Bringolf	Centre for Universal Design Australia Ltd., Australia
Yao Jen Chang	Chung Yuan Christian University, Taiwan, Republic of China
Mario Ciampi	National Research Council of Italy, Italy
Stuart Cunningham	Manchester Metropolitan University, UK
Georg Duftschmid	Medical University of Vienna, Austria
Stefano Federici	University of Perugia, Italy
David Fuschi	BRIDGING Consulting Ltd., UK
Alastair Gale	Loughborough University, UK
Ennio Gambi	Università Politecnica delle Marche, Italy
Janis Gogan	Bentley University, USA
Javier Gómez Escribano	Universidad Autónoma de Madrid, Spain
Jaakko Hakulinen	Tampere University, Finland
Tarja Heponiemi	Finnish Institute for Health and Welfare, Finland
Roberto Hornero	University of Valladolid, Spain
David Isern	Universitat Rovira i Virgili, Spain
Eila Järvenpää	Aalto University, Finland
Jeongeun Kim	Seoul National University, Korea, Republic of
Peter Kokol	University of Maribor, Slovenia
Stathis Konstantinidis	University of Nottingham, UK
Antonio Lanatà	University of Florence, Italy
Mikel Larrea	Universidad del País Vasco, Spain
Jin Luo	University of West London, UK

Heikki Lyytinen	University of Jyväskylä, Finland
Maurice Mars	University of KwaZulu-Natal, South Africa
Cezary Mazurek	Poznań Supercomputing and Networking Center, Poland
Elvis Mazzoni	University of Bologna, Italy
Kathleen McCoy	University of Delaware, USA
Hamid Mcheick	University of Quebec at Chicoutimi, Canada
René Meier	Lucerne University of Applied Sciences and Arts, Switzerland
Iosif Mporas	University of Hertfordshire, UK
Maurice Mulvenna	Ulster University, UK
Amit Nanavati	IBM Research, India
Marko Periša	University of Zagreb, Croatia
Marco Porta	Università degli Studi di Pavia, Italy
Amon Rapp	University of Torino, Italy
Ulrich Reimer	Eastern Switzerland University of Applied Sciences, Switzerland
Sreela Sasi	Gannon University, USA
Andreas Schrader	Universität zu Lübeck, Germany
Jitae Shin	Sungkyunkwan University, Korea, Republic of
Oh-Soon Shin	Soongsil University, Korea, Republic of
Josep Silva	Universitat Politècnica de València, Spain
Telmo Silva	University of Aveiro, Portugal
Åsa Smedberg	Stockholm University, Sweden
Susanna Spinsante	Università Politecnica delle Marche, Italy
Kostas Stathis	Royal Holloway, University of London, UK
Taro Sugihara	Tokyo Institute of Technology, Japan
Andrea Vitaletti	Sapienza University of Rome, Italy
Meng Wong	National Institute of Education, Singapore
George Xylomenos	Athens University of Economics and Business, Greece
Evi Zouganeli	Oslo Metropolitan University, Norway

Additional Reviewer

Rita Oliveira	University of Aveiro, Portugal

Invited Speakers

Raian Ali	Hamad Bin Khalifa University, Qatar
Maurice Mulvenna	Ulster University, UK
Jan Gulliksen	KTH Royal Institute of Technology, Sweden

Contents

On-Line Retrieval of Health Information Based on Language Complexity, Information Customization and Information Quality

Marco Alfano[3,4]([✉]) [iD], Biagio Lenzitti[1] [iD], Davide Taibi[2] [iD], and Markus Helfert[3] [iD]

[1] Dipartimento di Matematica e Informatica, Università di Palermo, Palermo, Italy
biagio.lenzitti@unipa.it
[2] Istituto per le Tecnologie Didattiche, Consiglio Nazionale delle Ricerche, Palermo, Italy
davide.taibi@itd.cnr.it
[3] Lero, Maynooth University, Maynooth, Co. Kildare, Ireland
{marco.alfano,markus.helfert}@lero.ie
[4] Anghelos Centro Studi sulla Comunicazione, Palermo, Italy

Abstract. A patient, nowadays, acquires on-line health information mainly by means of a search engine. Generic search engines have been shown to be limited and unsatisfactory, at times, because of their generic searches that overload users with the amount of results. Moreover, they are not able to provide customized information to different types of users. At the same time, specific search engines mostly work on medical literature and provide extracts from medical journals that are mainly useful for medical researchers and experts. As a consequence, the found health information may or may not help a user (mainly a non-expert one) for a full comprehension of what he/she is looking for (e.g., a condition, a therapy or a drug). This may negatively affect his/her empowerment process and the interaction with healthcare professionals such as doctors. This work presents a custom search engine, FACILE, that allows to overcome the limitations discussed above by facilitating finding and comprehension of on-line information and thus positively affecting the empowerment process and communication/interaction with healthcare professionals. A user, both a medical expert or non-expert, can specify his/her information requirements in terms of language level, specific information searched, and information quality. FACILE will provide the links to the web pages that comply with such requirements. In particular, FACILE will provide links to web pages with different language levels (simple or complex) and, for each link, the response page will show the requested specific information (condition, therapy, drug, etc.) and a graphical indication (0–5 stars) of the information quality.

Keyword: Digital health patient empowerment · Patient-doctor communication · Health information seeking · User requirements · Structured data · Search engine

1 Introduction

Health empowerment of people and communities is part of the "Framework on integrated people-centred health services" of WHO [1] and drives towards a paradigm shift

© Springer Nature Switzerland AG 2021
M. Ziefle et al. (Eds.): ICT4AWE 2020, CCIS 1387, pp. 1–20, 2021.
https://doi.org/10.1007/978-3-030-70807-8_1

on the relation between patients/citizens and health. Empowered people/patients have the necessary knowledge, skills, attitudes and self-awareness about their condition to understand their lifestyle and treatment options, make informed choices about their health and have control over the management of their condition/health in their daily life [2–9].

The acquisition of medical/health information is a basic step in the empowerment process and the main source of health/medical information is, nowadays, the Web [10–13]. Search engines are the main tools used to retrieve information from the Web [14, 15]. However, generic search engines do not make any distinction among the users and overload them with a huge amount of information that is often outdated and of poor quality. Moreover, the Web is full of information not easily understandable by users such as patients/citizens because they lack a specific expertise in the health domain. Specialized search engines (PubMed[1] or Cochrane Library[2]) mainly work on medical literature and are quite complex for generic users, and especially the elderly ones. Finally, specialized health/medical websites (e.g., WebMD[3], MedlinePlus[4], or Health on Net Foundation Select[5]) are mainly built by hand so presenting a limited and often outdated amount of information (compared to what is available on the Web). In addition, they are often not free.

The retrieval of health information from the Web requires a communication process between a user and a search engine. Notice that a "complete" communication process, usually, entails different levels of communication. Many communication models exist in the literature and a very famous model (if not the most famous) is the one introduced by Morris in relation to his theory of signs [16]. It is made up of three levels, i.e., *syntactic, semantic,* and *pragmatic* and it has been used in several works dealing with human communication [17–19]. Shannon and Weaver looked at other aspects of communication and presented a mathematical theory of communication that is focused on information transmission [20]. Even though they were mainly dealing with the technical aspects of communication, they introduced other two levels above the *technical* one, i.e., the *semantic* and *effectiveness* levels, that are influenced by the *technical* level.

This *syntactic-semantic-pragmatic* communication model can be used, in principle, for human-to-human communication (e.g., Patient-Doctor) whereas the *technical-semantic-effectiveness* communication model can be used for human-to-machine communication (e.g., Patient-Web), as shown in Fig. 1. Unfortunately, these communication models are not fully used for both Patient-Doctor communication (very often doctors use a technical language that is too complex for patients) and Patient-Web communication (a search engine only works at the technical level by retrieving web-page addresses based on user keywords). Even worse, the two communication processes often aim to opposite directions. In fact, when a patient looks for medical information on the Web before seeing a doctor, this often leads to the infamous quarrel between patients and doctors during the visit [21]. The Patient-Doctor and Patient-Web communication processes are,

---

[1] https://pubmed.ncbi.nlm.nih.gov/.

[2] https://www.cochranelibrary.com/.

[3] https://www.webmd.com/.

[4] https://medlineplus.gov/.

[5] https://www.hon.ch/HONselect/index.html.

in this case, contrasting each other and, surely, are not coherently contributing to the overall comprehension process of health conditions, treatments, etc., by patients.

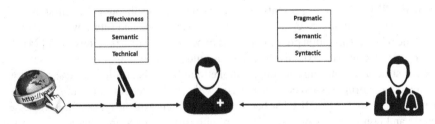

Fig. 1. Patient-Web and Patient-Doctor communication models.

Interestingly enough, the two models have been connected by [22] and an equivalence between the terms at the three levels has been established, in practice. We can then consider an *integrated* communication model that presents the following levels (with the *semantic* term that has been associated with *meaning* as indicated in [23]):

- **Pragmatic-Effectiveness:** How effectively does the received information affect behaviour?
- **Semantic-Meaning:** How precisely is the meaning conveyed?
- **Syntactic-Technical:** How accurately can the information be transmitted?

The objective is then to allow Patient-Web and Patient-Doctor communication to harness the three levels of the communication model and to aim to the same direction for the benefit of the person/patient. As seen above, the communication/interaction between a human user and a generic search engine only involves the syntactic-technical level by retrieving Web-page addresses (URLs) based on the keyword(s) specified by the user. A generic search engine has not been designed to understand user specific requirements (in his/her own language) and, thus, it is only able to provide the user with generic information leaving him/her with the task of selecting, understanding and using the retrieved information (semantic and pragmatic part of the communication process). Therefore, non-medical experts can be overwhelmed with the results and experience great difficulties in the comprehension and use of the found information. This, in turn, reflects on their ability to have a "true" two-way communication with their doctors because, for example, they do not have a complete understanding of their medical conditions (semantic level)–when they do not misunderstand them–and then they are unable to make shared and informed decisions (pragmatic level).

This work presents the characteristics and use of a custom search engine, FACILE, that has been created to satisfy the user information needs and overcome the communication challenges confronted during the search process. FACILE allows a user to specify his/her information requirements in a simple way. It, then, retrieves tailored Web information by exploiting the Web semantic capabilities provided by schema.org structured data. By doing so, FACILE provides the "right" amount of Web content, without overwhelming the user, and in a language that he/she can easily understand. This positively affects person/patient comprehension of conditions, treatment alternatives, etc.

and, ultimately, facilitates, his/her empowerment process and communication with medical professionals. The paper is organized as follows. Section 2 presents the principles and main characteristics of FACILE. Section 3 presents the implementation details and use of FACILE. Section 4 presents some experimental results and a discussion of the obtained results. Finally, Sect. 5 presents some conclusions and future work.

Some of the information presented in this paper is based on a previous work [24]. The present paper, however, extends the previous study by adopting a newer dataset, from 2019, of structured data and extracting a higher number of health-lifesci.schema.org and schema.org quadruples so to provide the user with a richer set of information. Moreover, the mapping model of FACILE has been improved to separate the types of users (medical experts and non-experts) and provide them with differentiated information in terms of language level and specific information. Furthermore, the FACILE interface has been completely redesigned in terms of usability and the customized information, as well as the quality information, is shown to favor user comprehension. Finally, FACILE principles and characteristics have been revised and are explained in more details and some new experimental results are presented to back FACILE effectiveness.

2   FACILE Principles and Characteristics

FACILE is a custom search engine specifically designed to facilitate the search of health information online by allowing users to specify their requirements during the search. In what follows we present its main principles and characteristics.

2.1   Identification of Requirements of On-Line Health Information Seekers

The identification of the main user requirements when searching for health information on the Web has been carried out in [4] by analysing the works presented in [14, 15, 25–29]. This literature review, although limited, has consistently shown the following main requirements by on-line health information seekers:

– Language complexity;
– Information classification/customization;
– Information quality (mainly intended as information trustworthiness).

The FACILE search engine has been developed, based on these requirements by exploiting the semantic features of the Web and particularly those related to structured data and schema.org with particular reference to its health-lifesci extension.

2.2   Use of schema.org and Health-Lifesci Structured Data

As said above, we have investigated how to leverage structured data to find suitable Web pages that satisfy the requirements of on-line health information seekers. To this end, we have exploited the semantic information available in the Web and, in particular, the one provided by schema.org[6], an initiative funded by some major Web players, that

---

[6] https://www.schema.org/.

aims to create, maintain, and promote schemas for structured data on the Internet. For the scope of the present work, we have considered the health-lifesci[7] extension that presently contains 80 types, 162 properties and 125 enumeration values related to the health/medical field.

We have performed an analysis of the health-lifesci elements using the data made available by the Web Data Commons initiative. The Web Data Commons (WDC) [30] contain all Microformat, Microdata and RDFa (Resource Description Framework in Attributes) data extracted from the open repository of Web crawl data named Common Crawl (CC). The data used in this work have been released in November 2019. The whole dataset contains about 2.5 billion pages and about 38.1% of them contain structured data.

The dataset dump, used in our study, consists of 44.2 billion RDF quadruples. These are sequences of RDF terms in the form {s, p, o, u}, where {s, p, o} represents a statement consisting of subject, predicate, object, while u represents the URI of the document from which the statement has been extracted. From the whole dataset, we have selected the subset containing one or more of the 367 elements (types, properties, and enumeration values) of health-lifesci.schema.org. The obtained subset contains 125,920,198 quadruples.

As a first step, the extracted quadruples have been directly inserted into a DB table with a size of around 16 GB. Next, in order to make the consultation of this table faster and more efficient, an indexing process has been carried out by replacing the four elements of the quadruple with the indexes of four indexed tables, one for each element.

2.3 Mapping Health Information Seeker Requirements to schema.org Elements

When speaking of on-line health information seekers, we can, mainly, consider two classes of users:

- Non experts (e.g., patients or citizens);
- Experts (e.g., physicians or medical researchers).

These two categories have different requirements, that can be connected to the language complexity and the other user requirements presented above. It is, then, important to understand which schema.org elements can be mapped to the user requirements to use the structured data present in the Web and deliver tailored information to the user.

Language Complexity. In relation to the language-complexity requirement, health-lifesci.schema.org includes the *MedicalAudience* element that indicates whether the content is more suitable for a non-expert (*Patient* type) or an expert (*Clinician* and *MedicalResearcher* types) [31]. A preliminary analysis of the dataset containing the health.life-sci.schema.org quadruples has shown that only a small part (around 5%) contains one or more *Patient, Clinician* or *MedicalResearcher* schema.org elements. Thus, by taking only those URLs, we would limit the search because most web pages containing health/medical schema.org structured information would not be considered. Moreover, the fact that a web page contains a *Patient* schema.org element does not

---

[7] https://health-lifesci.schema.org/.

necessarily indicate that those pages have a simpler language but only that they are targeted to patients (probably because of the page content). The same applies to the web pages that contain *Clinician* or *MedicalResearcher* schema.org elements that do not necessarily indicate the language used is complex.

In another work [31], we have measured the language complexity levels of the URLs containing *Patient*, *Clinician* or *MedicalResearcher* elements and generalized the analysis to URLs that do not contain any of these elements. To this end, we have analysed the English and non-empty web pages (around 50%) of the *Patient*, *Clinician* and *MedicalResearcher* subsets and, for each web page, we have computed its language complexity level. This has been done by computing the 'term familiarity index' [31–33] of each term found in the page (number of Google results) and then calculating the average for the page.

The experimental results, presented in [31], show that the web pages targeted to *Patient*, present, on average, a much higher term familiarity index whereas the web pages targeted to *Clinician* and *MedicalResearcher* present, on average, a lower term familiarity index. This kind of equivalence has convinced us to provide non-experts with URLs presenting a high term familiarity index (and thus a simpler terminology) and experts with URLs presenting a low term familiarity index (and thus a more complex terminology). By doing so, we are able to rank all URLs on the base of the FACILE language level, i.e., simple for non-experts and complex for experts. Moreover, coherently with the *MedicalAudience* schema.org representation, URLs containing a *Patient* schema.org element will be ranked higher for non experts whereas URLs containing *Clinician* or *MedicalResearcher* schema.org elements will be ranked higher for experts.

Information Customization. In order to proceed with a customization of information for the users, we have preliminarily investigated what type of health/medical information is primarily searched on the Web, such as medical conditions, therapies and drugs [10, 11, 14]. We have then verified that this type of information appears amongst the most recurring health-lifesci.schema.org elements to have enough data to be processed by FACILE and provide an effective information classification/customization. At the end of this process, we have selected the following health.life-sci.schema.org elements for creating the classification of Web pages (the definitions are taken from https://health-lif esci.schema.org/):

- *MedicalCondition*, indicates any condition of the human body that affects the normal functioning of a person, whether physically or mentally.
- *MedicalTherapy*, indicates a medical intervention designed to prevent, treat, and cure human diseases and medical conditions.
- *Drug*, indicates a chemical or biologic substance, used as a medical therapy, that has a physiological effect on an organism.
- *MedicalClinic*, indicates a hospital or a medical school.
- *MedicalCode*, provides a code for a medical entity.
- *MedicalScholarlyArticle*, indicates a medical article.

Note that the information on conditions, therapies, drugs, and hospitals can be of interest to both non-experts and experts whereas the information on codes and medical articles are more technical and so mainly indicated for medical experts. Therefore, we have decided to consider the first four elements for non-experts and all six elements for experts.

Information Quality. The health-lifesci.schema.org elements, being focused on the health/medical field, did not provide us with elements that can be immediately used for evaluating the information quality. Instead, by analyzing the literature [34–36], we found that the more general schema.org was able to provide some of those elements. We have selected *author, publisher, reviewedBy* and *recognizingAuthority* schema.org elements as an indication of reliability and *dateCreated, dateModified, datePublished* and *lastReviewed* schema.org elements as an indication of timeliness.

Note that, in principle, on-line health information seekers have the same requirements on the quality information irrespective of them being medical experts or not. Consequently, we have selected the same schema.org elements for providing information quality to both non-experts and experts.

Mapping Table. The above considerations about language complexity, information customization and information quality have led us to create a mapping between the user requirements and the schema.org elements for the non-expert and expert user categories. This mapping expands the one presented in [4, 24] and is reported in Table 1.

These schema.org elements are used by FACILE to retrieve Web pages and extract information based on the user specific requirements. As we will show in the next sections, by using FACILE, users can easily and quickly find the right amount of information that is reliable and, in a language suitable to their health literacy level, in full compliance with the three levels of the communication model presented above.

Table 1. Mapping between user requirements and schema.org elements for the "non-expert" and "expert" user categories.

	Language complexity	Information customization	Information quality
Non-expert	Simple *- High Term Familiarity*	*- MedicalCondition* *- MedicalTherapy* *- Drug* *- MedicalClinic*	Reliability: *- author* *- publisher* *- reviewedBy* *- recognizingAuthority* Timeliness: *- dateCreated* *- dateModified* *- datePublished* *- lastReviewed*

(continued)

Table 1. (*continued*)

	Language complexity	Information customization	Information quality
Expert	Complex - *Low Term Familiarity*	- *MedicalCondition* - *MedicalTherapy* - *Drug* - *MedicalClinic* - *MedicalCode* - *MedicalScholarlyArticle*	Reliability: - *author* - *publisher* - *reviewedBy* - *recognizingAuthority* Timeliness: - *dateCreated* - *dateModified* - *datePublished* - *lastReviewed*

3   FACILE Implementation and Use

The mapping between user requirements and schema.org elements, shown in the previous Section, has been used to build FACILE in order to provide experts and non-experts with the proper Web contents in terms of language complexity, information customization and information quality. It completes the previous versions of the system, the first one considering only the language level [31] and the second one taking into account only the information customization and quality [24]. Moreover, the algorithm used to provide the custom information has been completely revised with respect to the previous versions. Fig. 2 shows the user interface of the FACILE search engine for non-experts (a) and experts (b). FACILE is available at the address https://cohealth.lero.ie/facile.

The user interface includes a simple text input, like that of a generic search engine, where the user can insert the term(s) to be searched. Moreover, the user can filter the results to get more focused information by specifying his/her requirements in terms of language level, specific information required and information quality. The *simple* language level is recommended for non-experts whereas the *complex* language level is recommended for experts. Non-experts can select specific information by checking one or more of the four items reported in Fig. 2a whereas experts can choose one or more of the six items reported in Fig. 2b. Finally, the "Show Quality Information" switch, acts on the quality user requirement, for both types of users, and provides a measure of the quality of the web pages by evaluating the schema.org parameters reported in Table 1 (when available). In what follows we provide further details on the implementation and use of FACILE.

3.1   Language Level and Ranking Algorithm

After having inserted the quadruples into the database, as seen in Sect. 2.2, the English web pages have been analysed. For each web page, the *Term Frequency* of each word (not considering the stop words, i.e., the most common words) has been calculated together with its *Term Familiarity* (by using a Google™ API which returns the number of google results for a term). Depending on the selected language level, simple or complex, FACILE ranks the found URLs according to the following ranking formulas:

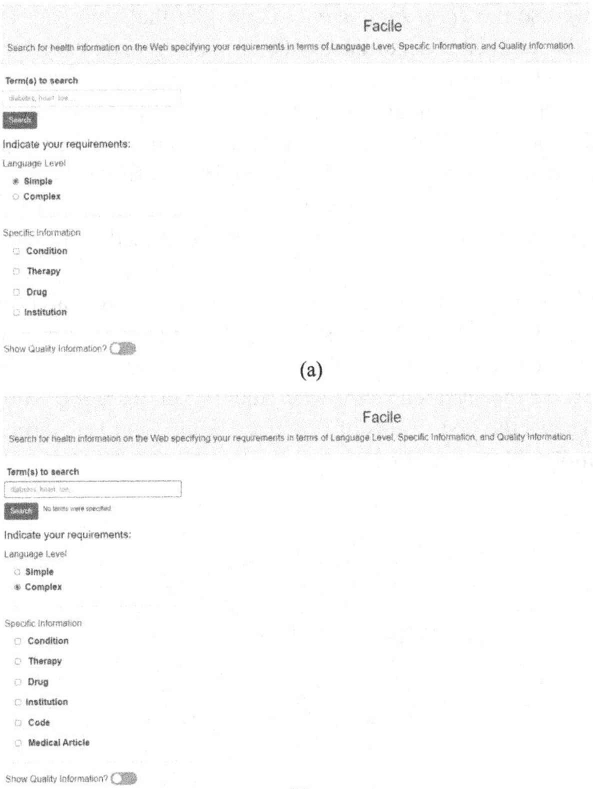

(a)

(b)

Fig. 2. FACILE user interface.

Simple Language.

$$R = \alpha * (Term\_Frequency/Max\_Term\_Frequency) + (1-\alpha) * \\ (Page\_Familiarity\_Index)/Max\_Familiarity\_Index) \tag{1}$$

Complex Language.

$$R = \alpha * (Term\_Frequency/Max\_Term\_Frequency) + (1-\alpha) * \\ (1 - Page\_Familiarity\_Index / Max\_Familiarity\_Index) \tag{2}$$

Where:

- *Term_Frequency* is the number of occurrences of the keyword(s) in the page divided by the document length;
- *Max_Term_Frequency* is the maximum of *Term_Frequency* of the keyword(s) in all found Web pages;
- *Page_Familiarity_Index* is the page familiarity, i.e., the mean of the term familiarity indexes of the Web page;
- *Max_Familiarity_Index* is the maximum page familiarity of all found Web pages.
- α allows to differently weigh the term frequency and page familiarity.

Notice that we use the *Term Frequency* to consider that web pages have different lengths and then the number of occurrences of a term can greatly vary. Notice, also, that the simple-language formula is a weighted combination of the *Term-Frequency* percentage and *Term-Familiarity* percentage because we want to find meaningful pages (i.e., with a high number of occurrences of the searched item) but with the simplest language. The complex-language formula is a weighted combination of the *Term-Frequency* percentage and (1 − *Term-Familiarity* percentage) because we want to find meaningful pages (i.e., with a high number of occurrences of the searched item) but with the most complex/technical language.

We have made some preliminary experiments with the weight and found out that a value of $\alpha = 0.4$ provided us with the best results in terms of correspondence between the intended audience and the provided Web pages. For example, Fig. 3 shows the first results of FACILE for the "asthma" term when the user chooses the "simple" language level and Fig. 4 shows the first results of FACILE for the "asthma" term when the user chooses the "complex" language level.

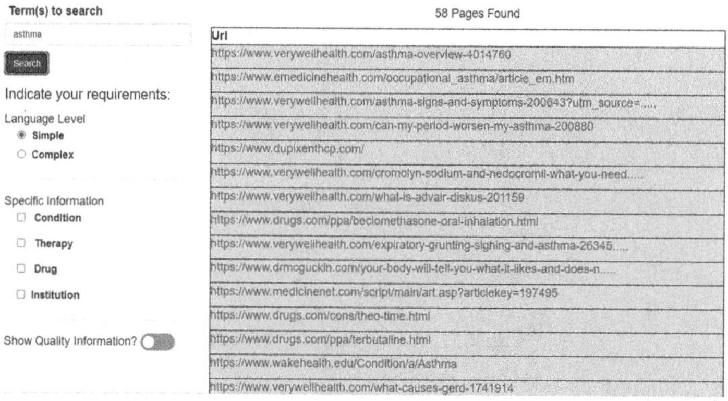

Fig. 3. FACILE results for "simple" language level.

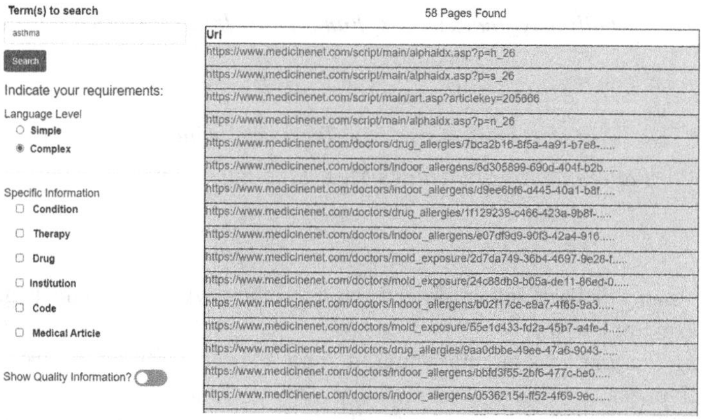

Fig. 4. FACILE results for "complex" language level.

3.2 Information Customization

As shown in Fig. 2, the user has the possibility to select which specific information he/she is interested in through checkboxes that can be easily selected by a user with no specific knowledge, because they indicate common terms in the health domain. More than one checkbox can be checked at the same time. FACILE will extract the custom information by using the mapping of Table 1 and will provide the following results:

- **Condition (for Non-experts and Experts):** It will present the pages that contain a description of a medical condition and the values of the properties related to the *MedicalCondition* schema.org element. In order not to overwhelm the user with information on the response page, FACILE will only show the values of the *name, alternateName*, and *description* properties.
- **Therapy (for Non-experts and Experts):** It will present the pages that contain information about a therapy and the values of the properties related to the *MedicalTherapy* schema.org element. In order not to overwhelm the user with information on the response page, FACILE will only show the values of the *name, alternateName, description, potentialAction,* and *contraindication* properties.
- **Drug (for Non-experts and Experts):** It will present the pages that contain the information about a medicine and the values of the properties related to the *Drug* schema.org element. In order not to overwhelm the user with information on the response page, FACILE will only show the values of the *name, nonPropietaryName, activeIngredient, description,* and *prescriptionStatus* properties.
- **Institution (for Non-experts and Experts):** It will present the pages that contain the institutions (e.g., hospitals) that deal with a medical condition and the values of the properties related to the *MedicalClinic* schema.org element. In order not to overwhelm the user with information on the response page, FACILE will only show the values of the *alternateName, description, hasMap, image, telephone,* and *email* properties.
- **Code (for Experts):** It will present the pages that contain the code of a medical condition and the values of the properties related to the *MedicalCode* schema.org element. In order not to overwhelm the user with information on the response page, FACILE will only show the values of the *name, alternateName, description, code, codeValue,* and *codingSystem* properties. The *code*, together with the *codingSystem*, can be used to look on specialized websites to find a specific condition/part of the body/therapy/drug, or other useful information.
- **MedicalScholarlyArticle (for Experts):** It will present the pages that contain information about medical scholarly articles and the values of the properties related to the *MedicalScholarlyArticle* schema.org element. In order not to overwhelm the user with information on the response page, FACILE will only show the values of the *description, publicationType, url, abstract, author, creator, dateCreated, datePublished, editor, headline,* and *sameAs* properties.

Fig. 5 shows the first results of FACILE for the "asthma" term (with simple language) when the user selects the Condition, Drug and Institution fields of the specific information.

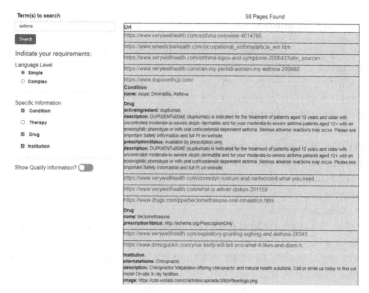

Fig. 5. FACILE results (simple language) with specific information checked.

Fig. 6 shows the first results of FACILE for the "asthma" term (with complex language) when the user selects the Medical-Article field of the specific information.

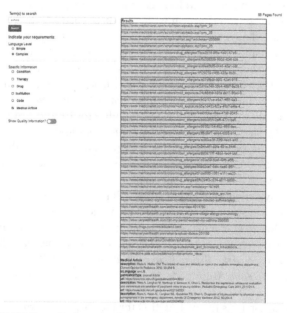

Fig. 6. FACILE results (complex language) with specific information checked.

3.3 Information Quality

The quality of the web pages provided by FACILE is evaluated in terms of reliability and timeliness by checking the presence of the schema.org elements reported in Table 1. To provide the user with a value and a visual indication about the information quality of the page, we have thought to provide each element with a weight that considers its relative importance. Considering some analysed literature [34–36], we have decided to assign different weights to the elements for a total of 10. As a first step, we have decided to assign 2/3 of the weights to Reliability and 1/3 of the weights to Timeliness because we want to value more reliability over timeliness. As a second step, we have assigned the following weights to the information quality schema.org elements:

- Reliability:
  - *author*   1
  - *publisher*   1.5
  - *reviewedBy*   1.5
  - *recognizingAuthority*   2.5   (Tot. 6.5)

- Timeliness:
  - *dateCreated*   0.5
  - *dateModified*   1.5
  - *datePublished*   0.5
  - *lastReviewed*   1   (Tot. 3.5)

Thus, for each web page, FACILE checks the presence of one or more quality-information elements and sums up the related weights. In order to provide the user with a direct visual information FACILE divides the result by two, rounds it to the whole or the half, and transforms the obtained number in stars so to provide each page with a number of stars that ranges between 0 and 5, with steps of half a star. Fig. 7 shows the first results of FACILE for the "asthma" term (with simple language and specific information checked) when the "Show Quality Information" switch is turned on.

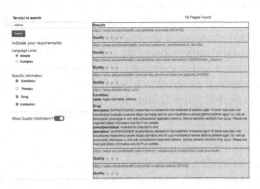

Fig. 7. FACILE results with "show quality information" switched on.

Notice that by clicking on the quality stars, the specific information-quality data will be shown (Fig. 8) so that the user will have the possibility to directly analyse them.

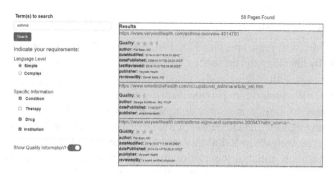

Fig. 8. Quality information details obtained by clicking on the quality stars.

4   Experimental Results and Discussion

FACILE, as shown in the previous Sections, has been designed and implemented to be used by different user typologies, i.e., medical experts or non-experts and we have executed some tests to evaluate its effectiveness and usefulness.

FACILE can be used as any other search engine by inserting any keyword(s) on the text input (Fig. 2). It will then rank the results in terms of the language level: simple (by default), as shown in Fig. 3, or complex, as shown in Fig. 4. For example, the first result of Fig. 3 presents a term familiarity of 3.53 million whereas the first result of Fig. 4 presents a term familiarity of 0.88 million. This clearly indicates how FACILE can separate pages with simple language from the ones with complex language. It already shows how FACILE outperforms a generic search engine in terms of providing web results with different language levels since a generic search engine is not able to provide such kind of responses.

The effectiveness of FACILE can further be appreciated when the specific-information fields are checked. In the example of Fig. 5, the condition, drug and institution fields are checked and this information is immediately shown in the response page for the web pages that contain it. This allows a user to save time by immediately finding the specific information he/she is looking for without the need of going through the content of the web pages. He/she will examine the complete content of the web pages only if he/she needs further information. In the example of Fig. 6, an expert user has checked the Medical-Article field and immediately gets a list of scientific articles with the related links. In this case, the user does not even need to browse the web page because the links to the articles, on the response page, allow him/her to directly go the articles of interest.

If the user switches on the "Show Quality Information" button, the quality of the web page is visually shown as a number of stars (0–5, Fig. 7), immediately providing the user with an information on the page trustworthiness. Nevertheless, if the user wants more detailed information about the quality, this information will be shown by clicking on the quality stars (Fig. 8). Notice that, the fact that a web page has a small number of stars (or no stars at all), does not necessarily imply that the information quality of the page is low and that the page is not trustworthy, but only that the chosen schema.org elements are not present. Thus, in general, a user is encouraged first to look at the web pages with a high number of stars, because that means that the page is of good quality, and then at the web pages with a low number of stars if they present other elements of interest.

To complete the evaluation of FACILE, we have run some experiments that compute the term familiarity of the web pages with simple and complex language levels. We have used six of the most searched diseases in Google™[8] and, in particular, three common terms (diabetes, depression, and anxiety) and three less common terms (yeast infection, psorias and lyme disease). The first ten results of each search have been considered and, for each group, the average familiarity index has been computed. Fig. 9 shows the results of this analysis (term familiarity is expressed in million). As expected, the web pages with a simple language level present a higher term familiarity than the web pages with the complex language level. More interesting is the fact that there is a clear separation between the familiarity indexes of the two categories even though the familiarity indexes of the web pages with simple-language levels are quite constant and the familiarity indexes of the web pages with complex-language levels present more differences. This appears more evident for the familiarity indexes of the less common terms (more technical) that present, in general, a higher term familiarity. This can be attributed to the fact that the common terms have a higher number of web pages and then a clearer separation between pages targeted to medical experts and non-experts whereas the less common terms have a lower number of web pages and they appear more targeted to non-experts (considering their higher familiarity indexes). Further experiments are undoubtedly needed to better understand FACILE behavior in these cases.

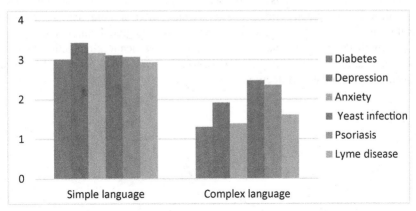

Fig. 9. Average familiarity indexes (in million) of most searched health diseases in Google™.

Although FACILE can still be improved and more experiments are undoubtedly needed, its principles and practical use show how it complies with the three-level communication model presented in the Introduction. In particular:

Syntactic-Technical: FACILE presents the same retrieval capabilities as a generic search engine and, as such, it allows the user to search for health information on the Web (although it restrains the search to the Web structured data) and provides the requested information as any generic search engine does.

---

[8] https://www.beckershospitalreview.com/quality/most-commonly-googled-diseases.html.

Semantic-Meaning: The translation capability of FACILE (mapping model) allows the user to specify his/her requirements in simple terms. FACILE "understands" such requirements and translates them into schema.org elements to extract the proper information from the Web (communication phase: from user to FACILE). Moreover, the ability of FACILE, to retrieve Web pages with different language levels, allows the user to choose the pages with the preferred level (communication phase: from FACILE to user).

Pragmatic-Effectiveness: The response presented by FACILE has a pragmatic impact on the user by providing understandable, focused, and reliable Web results. The consequence is that a user (mainly non-expert/patient) is, overall, greatly facilitated in finding, understanding, and using health/medical information on the Web and then in his/her empowerment process. This, among others, facilitates the comprehension of his/her medical conditions and greatly increases his/her ability to communicate with medical professionals and make informed decisions. Moreover, the ability of FACILE to provide focused and customized information can also facilitate the task of medical professionals to accompany patients in their search of on-line health information.

Overall, FACILE provides the user with the possibility of filtering and re-ranking the Web results according to his/her specific requirements but it leaves the user fully in charge of his/her navigational path on the Web. In this way, a user can freely and simply choose what he/she needs in terms of health/medical information, in any moment, so to achieve his/her empowerment objectives and better communicate/interact with medical professionals. This allows, overall, to have an integrated communication with regards to both Patient-Web and Patient-Doctor communication/interaction (Fig. 10) that is aligned and overcomes, in practice, the well-known quarrel between doctors and patients discussed in the Introduction.

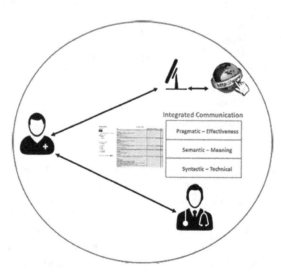

Fig. 10. FACILE integrated communication model.

Of course, an application that helps patient-doctor communication at the semantic level (helping mutual understanding) would be highly desirable. To this end, we have developed the SIMPLE application that translates the medical/technical terms of any text into lay terms, adding a short and simple explanation [37–39]. This helps users, mainly non-medical experts, to understand medical texts (e.g., medical reports) and then to better communicate with medical professionals. Notice that SIMPLE fully complies with the three-level communication model because it facilitates mutual understanding between patients and doctors (semantic level) and helps them in defining and reaching a specified objective (pragmatic level). The joint use of FACILE and SIMPLE allows, overall, a person/patient to communicate in the same (simple) way with both the Web, through FACILE, and a doctor, through SIMPLE, by fully exploiting the integrated communication model for human-to-machine and human-to-human communication.

5   Conclusions and Future Work

This work has presented a custom search engine, FACILE, that allows users (both medical experts and non-experts) to retrieve health information from the Web on the base of their specific requirements in terms of language level, information customization and information quality. FACILE maps those requirements into schema.org structured elements and retrieves the "right" and simple Web content without overwhelming the user as a generic search engine often does. This positively affects user understanding and use of health information and, therefore, the empowerment process and communication with healthcare professionals. Moreover, FACILE fully complies with the "integrated" three-levels communication model that allows a full interaction of a person/patient with both a machine (e.g., search engine) and another human (e.g., doctor).

The principles and first experimental results are satisfying and show FACILE potentialities even though, the used dataset (created with the 2019 structured data of Web Data Commons) has proven, sometimes, too limited in terms of provided results. Thus, we are in the process of adding the datasets of the previous years, such as the ones of 2018 and 2017, because the various datasets present some differences in terms of URLs and thus provide more data to experiment with. Furthermore, although the current version of FACILE is simple and intuitive and it has been widely improved with respect to its previous versions, we are in the process of running some tests with non-experts, such as elderly people, to evaluate their engagement level and understand the aspects that need further improvement. An evaluation of the reached empowerment level through FACILE is also important and we are in the process of running randomized control trials with patients with chronic conditions. The reached health literacy and empowerment levels will be measured because of the use of FACILE.

As a future work, we plan to analyse in more details the health-lifesci.schema.org elements to evaluate whether further customized information can be provided to the user but being always careful not to overwhelm him/her. We also plan to improve the information quality algorithm by considering the dates the web pages have been created, modified, published, and so on, beside just evaluating the presence of the related information. We also want to further develop the integrated communication model for improving the human-to-human and human-to-machine communication processes that underlie patient empowerment. For example, we plan to integrate the FACILE and SIMPLE applications to allow a person to use a single interface to find health information on-line and simplify it. Finally, we want to create a visual framework [40] that uses the retrieving capabilities of FACILE and translating capabilities of SIMPLE and allows easy creation of advanced health services, such as virtual assistants, for elderly people/patients.

Acknowledgements. This work was partially supported by the European Union's Horizon 2020 research and innovation programme under the Marie Skłodowska-Curie grant agreement No 754489 and by Science Foundation Ireland grant 13/RC/2094 with a co-fund of the European Regional Development Fund through the Southern & Eastern Regional Operational Programme to Lero, the Science Foundation Ireland Research Centre for Software, www.lero.ie.

References

1. World Health Organization (WHO). Framework on integrated, people-centred health services: Report by the Secretariat. World Health Assembly, (A69/39), pp. 1–12 (2016)
2. World Health Organization (WHO). (1998. Health promotion glossary. https://www.who.int/healthpromotion/about/HPR%20Glossary%201998.pdf
3. European Health Parliament. Patient Empowerment and Centredness (2017)
4. Alfano, M., Lenzitti, B., Taibi, D., Helfert, M.: Provision of tailored health information for patient empowerment: an initial study. In: Proceedings of the 20th International Conference on Computer Systems and Technologies (CompSysTech 2019). Association for Computing Machinery, New York, NY, USA, pp. 213–220 (2019). https://doi.org/10.1145/3345252.3345301
5. Herzog, M.A., Kubincová, Z., Han, P., Temperini, M. (eds.): Advances in web-based learning – ICWL 2019. LNCS, vol. 11841. Springer, Cham (2019). https://doi.org/10.1007/978-3-030-35758-0
6. Bodolica, V., Spraggon, M.: Toward patient-centered care and inclusive health-care governance: a review of patient empowerment in the UAE. Public Health **169**(971), 114–124 (2019)
7. Bravo, P., Edwards, A., Barr, P.J., Scholl, I., Elwyn, G., McAllister, M.: Conceptualising patient empowerment: a mixed methods study. BMC Health Serv. Res. **15**(1), 1–14 (2015)
8. Cerezo, P.G., Juvé-Udina, M.E., Delgado-Hito, P.: Concepts and measures of patient empowerment: a comprehensive review. Revista Da Escola de Enfermagem **50**(4), 667–674 (2016)
9. Fumagalli, L.P., Radaelli, G., Lettieri, E., Bertele', P., Masella, C.: Patient empowerment and its neighbours: clarifying the boundaries and their mutual relationships. Health Policy **119**(3), 384–394 (2015)
10. Pew Research Center. Health online (2013). https://www.pewinternet.org/2013/01/15/health-online-2013/
11. Taylor, H.: HI-Harris-Poll-Cyberchondrics. Harris Interactive (2010). https://theharrispoll.com/the-latest-harris-poll-measuring-how-many-people-use-the-internet-to-look-for-information-about-health-topics-finds-that-the-numbers-continue-to-increase-the-harris-poll-first-used-the-word-cyberch/
12. UK national statistics. Statistical bulletin: Internet Access. Office for National Statistics, 27 August 2010
13. Instituto Nacional de Estadística. Encuesta sobre Equipamiento y Uso de Tecnologías de la Información y Comunicación en los hogares (2010)

14. Pletneva, N., Vargas, A., Boyer, C.: D8.1.1. Requirements for the general public health search. Khresmoi Public Deliverable (2011)
15. Roberts, T.: Searching the internet for health information: techniques for patients to effectively search both public and professional websites. In: SLE Workshop at Hospital for Special Surgery Tips For Evaluating the Quality of Health, pp. 1–12 (2017)
16. Morris, C.W.: Foundations of the Theory of Signs. International Encyclopedia of Unified Science, vol. 1, no. 2. The University of Chicago Press, Chicago (1938)
17. Hahn, L.K., Paynton, S.T.: Survey of Communication Study (2014). https://en.wikibooks. org/wiki/Survey_of_Communication_Study
18. Cherry, C.: On Human Communication: A Review, A Survey, and A Criticism. M.I.T. Press, Cambridge (1966)
19. Johnson, F.C., Klare, G.R.: General models of communication research: a survey of the developments of a decade. J. Commun. 11(1), 13–26 (1961)
20. Shannon, C., Weaver, W.: The Mathematical Theory of Communications. University of Illinois Press, Urbana (1949)
21. Smith, T.: Exploring the characteristics of active health seekers, the thinking behind patient preferences, and the implications for patient-professional relationships. Qual. Safety Health Care 13(6), 474–477 (2004)
22. Carlile, P.: Transferring, translating and transforming: an integrative framework for managing knowledge across boundaries, organization. Science 15(5), 555–568 (2004)
23. Watzlawick, P., Beavin, J.B., Jackson, D.D.: Pragmatics of Human Communication: A Study of Interactional Patterns, Pathologies, and Paradoxes. Norton, New York (1967)
24. Alfano, M., Lenzitti, B., Taibi, D., Helfert, M.: Tailored retrieval of health information from the web for facilitating communication and empowerment of elderly people. In: Proceedings of the 6th International Conference on Information and Communication Technologies for Ageing Well and e-Health - Volume 1: ICT4AWE, pp. 205–216 (2020). https://doi.org/10. 5220/0009576202050216 ISBN 978-989-758-420-6
25. Banna, S., Hasan, H., Dawson, P.: Understanding the diversity of user requirements for interactive online health services. Int. J. Healthc. Technol. Manage. 15(3), 253–271 (2016)
26. Pian, W., Khoo, C.S.G., Chi, J.: Automatic classification of users' health information need context: logistic regression analysis of mouse-click and eye-tracker data. J. Med. Internet Res. 19(12), e424 (2017)
27. Pang, P.C.-I., Verspoor, K., Pearce, J., Chang, S.: Better health explorer: designing for health information seekers. In: OzCHI 2015 Proceedings of the Annual Meeting of the Australian Special Interest Group for Computer Human Interaction, pp. 588–597 (2015)
28. Keselman, A., Logan, R., Smith, C.A., Leroy, G., Zeng-Treitler, Q.: Developing informatics tools and strategies for consumer-centered health communication. J. Am. Med. Inf. Assoc. JAMIA 15(4), 473–483 (2008)
29. Ardito, S.C.: Seeking consumer health information on the internet. Online Searcher 37(4), 1–5 (2013). https://www.infotoday.com/OnlineSearcher/Articles/Medical-Digital/Seeking-Consumer-Health-Information-on-the-Internet-90558.shtml
30. Meusel, R., Petrovski, P., Bizer, C.: The webdatacommons microdata, RDFa and microformat dataset series. In: Mika, P. (ed.) The Semantic Web – ISWC 2014. LNCS, vol. 8796, pp. 277–292. Springer, Cham (2014). https://doi.org/10.1007/978-3-319-11964-9_18
31. Alfano, M., Lenzitti, B., Taibi, D., Helfert M.: Facilitating access to health Web pages with different language complexity levels. In: Proceedings of the 5th International Conference on Information and Communication Technologies for Ageing Well and e-Health (ICT4AWE 2019), 2–4 May 2019, Heraklion-Crete (2019)
32. Kloehn, N., et al.: Improving consumer understanding of medical text: development and validation of a new subsimplify algorithm to automatically generate term explanations in English and Spanish. J. Med. Internet Res. 20(8), e10779 (2018)

33. Leroy, G. et al.: Improving perceived and actual text difficulty for health information consumers using semi-automated methods. In: AMIA Annual Symposium Proceedings, pp. 522–531 (2012)
34. World Health Organization (WHO). Improving Data Quality: A Guide for Developing Countries, pp. 1–74 (2003). https://www.wpro.who.int/publications/docs/improving_data_quality.pdf
35. Eysenbach, G., Powell, J., Kuss, O., Sa, E.-R.: Empirical studies assessing the quality of health information for consumers on the world wide web: a systematic review. JAMA J. Am. Med. Assoc. **287**(20), 2691–2700 (2002). https://doi.org/10.1001/jama.287.20.2691
36. Jadad, A.R., Gagliardi, A.: Rating health information on the internet. JAMA **279**(8), 611 (1998)
37. Alfano, M., Lenzitti, B., Lo Bosco, G., Muriana, C., Piazza, T., Vizzini, G.: Design, development and validation of a system for automatic help to medical text understanding. Int. J. Med. Inf. (2020a). https://doi.org/10.1016/j.ijmedinf.2020.104109.
38. Alfano, M., Lenzitti, B., Lo Bosco, G., Taibi, D.: Development and Practical use of a medical vocabulary-thesaurus-dictionary for patient empowerment. In: Proceedings of ACM International Conference on Computer Systems and Technologies (CompSysTech 2018), Ruse (2018)
39. Alfano, M., Lenzitti, B., Lo Bosco, G., Perticone, V.: An automatic system for helping health consumers to understand medical texts. In: Proceedings of HEALTHINF 2015, Lisbon, pp. 622–627 (2015)
40. Alfano, M., Lenzitti, B., Lo Bosco, G., and Taibi, D.: A framework for opening data and creating advanced services in the health and social fields. In: Proceedings of ACM International Conference on Computer Systems and Technologies (CompSysTech 2016), Palermo (2016)

Emotions and Attitudes of Older Adults Toward Robots of Different Appearances and in Different Situations

Stephanie Lehmann[(✉)] [ID], Esther Ruf[ID], and Sabina Misoch[ID]

Institute for Ageing Research, OST Eastern Switzerland University of Applied Sciences, Rosenbergstrasse 59, 9001 St. Gallen, Switzerland
stephanie.lehmann@ost.ch

Abstract. The demographic change and the decrease of care personnel lead to the discussion to implement robots to support older adults. To ensure sustainable use, the solutions must be accepted. Technology Acceptance is dealt with in different models, but little attention has been paid to the emotions that older adults have toward service robots that support every day or care activities. The simulated robot study examined the positive and negative emotions and the attitudes of 142 older adults toward robots in different situations and with robots of different appearances. The situation influenced both emotions and attitudes. The older adults expressed more negative emotions and a more negative attitude in a care situation. In terms of appearance, less uncanniness and higher usage intention for the human-like and android robot were reported. The results contribute to a deeper understanding of robot acceptance and should be considered in the development of service robots for older adults in the future. Furthermore, the results should be validated in vivo with existing robots.

Keyword: Robot · Emotion · Attitude · Older adults

1 Background

1.1 Development of Technological Solutions to Support Older Adults

The development and use of technologies for older adults to support them and their caregivers are supported by various social trends. Above all, demographic change is leading to an increase in the elderly population [109]. In the European Union in 2018, the age group 65+ accounted for 19.7% of the total population with big differences between countries. Italy with 22.6% was at the highest end and Ireland with 13.8% at the lowest. What all countries have in common is the increase in the older population, especially as baby boomers reach retirement age [29]. Since many older adults wish to live independently in their familiar environment as long as possible [69], solutions are needed to support older adults in their private home. This can have a positive effect for their quality of life [100], which is in line with the aims of Ageing in Place [45]. Furthermore, solutions are needed to support nursing staff in care facilities, since the

© Springer Nature Switzerland AG 2021
M. Ziefle et al. (Eds.): ICT4AWE 2020, CCIS 1387, pp. 21–43, 2021.
https://doi.org/10.1007/978-3-030-70807-8_2

expected shortage of skilled nursing staff [121] is another major factor that is expected to lead to an increased use of technology and robotics.

Considering that worldwide more than two billion people will potentially need digital technologies by 2050 [122], these could support the well-being of older adults. It is assumed that robots will play an increasingly important role by maintaining the independence and well-being of older adults [92, 124]. They have proven benefits and can contribute to improving the quality of life of older people [9, 91], and they could contribute to maintaining the quality of care [10]. Robots offer the potential to support and relieve the burden on both older adults and their caregivers and they can also be used for prevention and rehabilitation purposes to avoid or reduce the need for assistance [42]. Promising areas of application of robots for social and daily healthcare of older adults are reported [2, 3]. The field of robotics in nursing is developing rapidly to meet the need for assistance in caregiving [65]. However, to realize the successful implementation of robots for older adults, user acceptance is essential, as so far little acceptance is reported for robots in care for older adults [114].

1.2   User Acceptance

Several models of Technology Acceptance portray the "Intention to Use" as an operationalization of acceptance. They vary in their differentiation, in the number of influencing factors, and in the field in which they were developed and tested. The basic Technology Acceptance Model (TAM) [21] has been developed further over time to the TAM 2 [111], TAM 3 [110] and the Unified Theory of Acceptance and Use of Technology model (UTAUT) [112]. Misoch, Pauli and Ruf [77] provide a critical discussion of Technology Acceptance models regarding their predictive power in relation to older adults. The Almere model [46] refers specifically to assistive robots for older adults. Extended to the context of service robots it developed into the Service Robot Acceptance Model (sRAM) [120].

Most of these models focus on cognitive (especially evaluative) and social factors. Emotions triggered by robots that support daily activities are considered rather globally (e.g. as "fear" dimension [124]) and unspecifically (e.g. as "emotional involvement" and "potential threat" [78]). Emotions of users are investigated at most concerning empathy with robots [95]. Some authors, such as Goher, Mansouri and Fadlallah [41] found the criterions "Ease of Use" and "Usefulness" to be the main factors for technology acceptance among older adults. However, in the study by De Graaf and Allouch [23], only the factor "Enjoyment" and not "Utility" indicates the actual use of a robot. Therefore, emotions of older adults should be given more emphasis in the consideration when interacting with a robot, as emotions and attitudes influence their reactions [14]. Although the integration of emotions in robot systems attempts to make robots empathetic, the emotional reactions of humans toward robots have not yet been explicitly investigated [94].

1.3   Emotions in Interaction Toward Robots Used for Older Adults

When robots perform tasks usually performed by humans and come into direct contact with humans for an intimate task it can evoke powerful emotions. Thus, embedding robots in new everyday situations can be emotionally challenging. Different types of robots can be used to support older adults and nursing staff. A distinction is often made between service type and companion type robots, although not all robots can be categorized strictly in either one of these two groups [16].

Robots referred to as service type robots are used as assistive devices with functionalities to support independent living. When it comes to the level of acceptance of these robots, studies usually focus on two aspects: types of social functions, that are important to accept the device in the living environment; how social functions can facilitate the usage of the device. Emotions that are triggered by these types of robots in older users were not the primary focus of research. It is expected that in assistive situations, the use of robots can lead to unclear expectations [19] and unrealistic ideas [8].

In contrast, emotions and reactions of older adults interacting with the second type, the so-called companion robots, are well studied [e.g. 1, 48, 72]. These companion robots are made to evoke explicitly positive emotions and are used as aids in therapy.

Nomura, Kanda and Suzuki [83] combine perspectives on societal attitudes and psychological reactions toward robots in their Negative Attitudes toward Robots Scale (NARS). In human-robot-interaction, communicative behavior is affected by the attitudes toward robots and anxiety related to robots [84].

1.4 Appearance of the Robot and Situation of Human-Robot Interaction

There are additional factors, such as characteristics of the robot or environmental factors, that can influence acceptance. The appearance of robots has been discussed as an important factor promoting or inhibiting acceptance [14, 35]. As robots are judged by users based on their appearance, it can trigger positive feelings toward the robot and thus lead to greater acceptance [49]. The appearance of a robot can be divided into different categories, for example in functional, zoomorphic, anthropomorphic, or cartoon-like [54]. With the idea that positive human-robot interaction is increased by human resemblance, humanoid robots are built in industrial contexts [e.g. 57]. Anthropomorphic robots also seem to reach higher levels of acceptance in settings with social interactions with a robot. Human-like shape and behavior have advantages when a close interaction between a robot and a human is necessary, and better performance in human-like tasks is assumed when a robot resembles a human [49]. Socially assistive robots that have human-like characteristics tend to promote acceptance and use [59]. However, there are varying findings when it comes to preferences on human-like robots. Broadbent [13] reports that older adults expressed a preference for non-humanlike robots, as they did not want them to replace humans. Other researchers found that older adults prefer discrete, small robots as well as human- or pet-like robots over large humanoid robots [15, 108, 123]. However, the "Uncanny Valley" hypothesis [80] states that the more human-like the appearance of the robot, the more accepted it is, unless it does not resemble a human too much. An abrupt decline in acceptance has been observed as soon as reaching a certain level of human resemblance in a robot. Android robots can be perceived as frightening when their movements are too mechanical and therefore do not match human appearance [68]. This gap in acceptance is subject of much debate, and mixed or inconsistent findings concerning the existence of the uncanny valley and its explanations are discussed [e.g. 47, 55, 66, 75, 104].

An important point regarding the appearance of a robot is that it cannot be considered independent to the situation of its use. Studies show that not only the appearance of the robot but also the situation in which a human-robot interaction takes place has a decisive influence on acceptance [22, 26, 39, 77]. The robot must fit the respective field of application or the task performed [13, 93], and the shape and capabilities of a robot should be congruent. Robots with a human-like appearance are attributed to have personality, emotions, and intentions [53]. This potential humanization leads to robots being considered as "trustworthy" and useful for trustful tasks.

Research from the fields of human-robot interaction (HRI), human-robot proxemics (HRP), and human-robot spatial interaction (HRSI) show that personal space is a major issue in human-robot interaction (for a summary see [63]), and the spatial area in which a robot moves during interaction is determined by the situation and its tasks. The robot should stay outside the intimate zone and within the personal or social zone of a person [56, 115]. If robots support daily activities of older adults, they are usually outside the intimate zone. This is different when robots support care activities which usually include touch in the intimate zone. Care workers were reserved toward robots in tasks that involve human touch [88].

Regarding the results from previous research, the following hypotheses have been examined in this study:

(1) Appearance of the robot: although inconsistent results in the literature, it is assumed that human-like to android robots will trigger more negative feelings in older adults.
(2) Situations when interacting with a robot: it is assumed that situations that require interaction in the intimate zone will evoke more negative feelings in older adults.

The present study aimed to investigate more comprehensively the emotions and attitudes of older adults toward robots of different appearances and in different situations. It aims to be a contribution to a better understanding of the acceptance of robots in this field, with the ability to lead to a sustainable use of robots. The study only refers to service type robots. According to the categorization of assistive robots for older adults by Broekens, Heerink, and Rosendal [16] the main function of service robots is to support daily activities. Companion robots (e.g. pet-like robots), whose main function is to improve health and psychological well-being, or other robot types, are not considered.

2   Methods

2.1   Design

A vignette methodology to collect emotions and attitudes toward robots was used. In vignettes, hypothetical situations are described, and participants are asked to put themselves into the hypothetical situation and to respond [6]. In human-robot interaction studies, this method has been used successfully and is a common methodology in psychology and sociology experiments [17, 31]. Video trials are used and regarded as a valid methodology [46].

Table 1. Study sample.

	N = 142 older adults
Age	73.2 years (SD = 6.1, range 58–87)
Gender	54.2% female
Marital status	71.1% married/living with partner
Nationality	97.9% Swiss
Education	65.5% tertiary level 23.2% secondary level 8.5% obligatory school education 0.7% no school leaving certificate
Living environment	98.6% private household
Household size	64.8% two-person household
Residential area	53.5% more rural
Interest in technology	21.8% very interested 50.0% interested 26.8% not interested 1.4% not interested at all
Technology experience	76.1% experience with technology use in professional life
Experience with robots	24.5% contact with a robot before

N = Number.

2.2 Participants

Via different existing networks of the Institute for Ageing Research (IAF), older adults who had to be German-speaking and aged over 60, were recruited in Eastern Switzerland. They were offered several possible study dates. A total of 11 study dates took place between September to December 2018 in three different Swiss cantons (St.Gallen, the Grisons, Lucerne). Table 1 shows the characteristics of the sample.

2.3 Measures

A questionnaire was developed to collect the emotions and attitudes of older adults toward robots. For emotion items, various existing scales were compiled based on a literature search. Table 2 shows the scales and basic emotions (overview in [86]) that were considered. Single emotions were added mentioned by older adults and the research team during a feasibility test in September 2017. A list with 79 positive, 12 neutral and 116 negative emotions was the result (see Fig. 1).

After this first compilation of a list with 207 emotion items, final items were selected separately by two researchers based on eight criteria (Table 3).

From the resulting list of 34 positive and 45 negative items, further individual items were sorted out based on content considerations when not fitting, being already covered by other items, or being too vague. The result was a two-page list with 30 positive

Table 2. Scales and basic emotions for questionnaire development.

Scale
German version of positive and negative affect schedule [12]
State-Trait-Anxiety Inventory [44]
SEK-ES–questionnaire for emotion-specific self-assessment of emotional competencies [25]
Jennifer Monathan "liking" questionnaire [79]
Emotional reactions to domestic robots [97]
Property list at the subscale level [52]
Feeling scale – Revised version (Bf-SR) [113]
Multidimensional state questionnaire (MDBF) [103]
Basic Emotions [4, 27, 37, 43, 50, 51, 71, 81, 85, 87, 89, 107, 118, 119]

Table 3. Criteria for item selection.

Criteria
(1) deletion of the category "neutral" because it was too unspecific
(2) ensuring comparability with other studies
(3) avoidance of doubled/too similar items
(4) same number of positive and negative items
(5) focus on "real" emotions and not "attitudes" or "evaluations"
(6) state emotions instead of trait emotions
(7) comprehensibility
(8) frequently occurring items

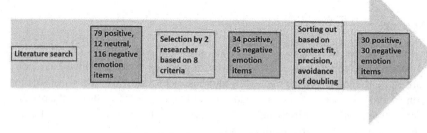

Fig. 1. Selection process of emotion items.

and 30 negative emotion items, presented as adjectives and displayed in random order. A dichotomous answer format ("rather yes" or "rather no") was chosen to allow the participants to fill in the questionnaire rapidly and easily. Figure 1 shows the selection process of the emotion items.

In addition, questions of robot acceptance were chosen based on the Almere model and the robot-acceptance questionnaire in the version by Heerink, Kröse, Evers and Wielinga [46]. Of the 41 items, six were selected which suited the context of the present study best. Two questions from the construct "Anxiety" (ANX), one from "Attitude toward Technology" (ATT), one from "Intention to Use" (ITU), one from "Perceived Ease of Use" (PEOU) and one question from "Perceived Usefulness" (PU) and translated into German and adapted. The answer format followed a five-point scale from 1 "do not at all agree" to 5 "agree completely".

Items following the recommendations from the review by Flandorfer [35] and items from previous questionnaires of the authors were chosen to collect sociodemographic data. Three further questions were included in the questionnaire which were described in the literature in the context of robots: Experience with technology from previous professional life ("Yes/No"), interest in technology on a four-level scale from "very interested" to "not at all interested" and the question "Have you ever dealt directly with a robot" from Nitto, Taniyama and Inagaki [82] to compare the Swiss population with the German and Japanese population.

Care was taken to ensure that the question formulations and answer categories of the questionnaire were age-appropriate (according to the recommendations of Lang [62]). Nine older adults (four men and five women 60+ years old) pretested the questionnaire. The final questionnaire consisted of four pages and could be completed in about 15 min.

2.4 Material

The vignette was presented in a video format supplemented with pictures of robots of different appearance. For the variation of the situation, two different video stimuli were selected. Each film showed a different situation of interaction with a robot. The video stimuli were tested beforehand in a feasibility test in September 2017. One situation showed an older woman in a retirement home sitting at a table with other older women, illustrating the service situation (S1). In this situation, the robot Care-O-bot 3 [36] moves toward the woman with a cup of water and then invites her to drink, which she does. The other situation showed a middle-aged bedridden woman, her arms and legs being washed by the robot Cody [40] without other people visible, illustrating the care situation (S2). Both video stimuli were cut to one minute in length, to accurately illustrate the relevant interaction. To avoid distractions through verbal descriptions they were shown without sound.

Because assistive robots have a wide range of different looks [22], pictures of robots with varying degrees of human resemblance were selected based on the most used classification of different authors: machine-like, mechanical-human-like, human-like, and android [24, 67, 116]. Pictures of high quality and that depicted meaningful representations in the context of nursing care for older adults were selected. The pictures were shown without product names of the robots. Pictures of the following robots were selected: Lio for machine-like appearance [30]; Kompai for mechanical-human-like appearance [106]; Romeo for human-like appearance [7]; Otonaroid for android appearance [76].

2.5 Procedure

Several participants took part in each of the 11 study sessions, which always followed the same pattern. After an introduction and explanation of the study, the participants were shown the first video (S1) and were asked to put themselves in this situation as if they were experiencing it themselves, imagining the appearance of the robot based on the picture given after the video. One of four images of a robot were given to the participants, resembling either machine-like (A1), mechanical-human-like (A2), human-like (A3) or android (A4). After the first completion of the questionnaire, the participants were given another picture of the robot and had to fill in another questionnaire. This procedure was repeated with the second video (S2) (Fig. 2 shows the procedure of the study sessions). According to a predetermined scheme ensuring all possible combinations occurred equally, each participant evaluated four randomly composed vignettes (see Table 4). Participants reported emotions and attitudes for each of the four vignettes with the questionnaire. Each participant was set apart in a classroom and filled in the questionnaire on his/her own and in silence. No joint discussion or audible comments were allowed during the study appointments.

Table 4. Combination of appearance and situations [96].

Appearance A	Situation S	
(A1–A4)	Service situation (S1)	Care situation (S2)
A1: machine-like	A1 × S1	A1 × S2
A2: mechanical-human-like	A2 × S1	A2 × S2
A3: human-like	A3 × S1	A3 × S2
A4: android	A4 × S1	A4 × S2

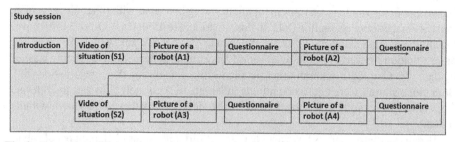

Fig. 2. Procedure of the study sessions. Order of presentation of one of the four pictures of a robot (A1–A4) varied.

2.6 Analysis

For evaluation, the IBM SPSS Statistics 26 program was used. After manually entering the data, a 5% check of the sample, quality control, and data cleansing were carried out.

The 30 positive and the 30 negative emotions were taken together to build a sum score for positive emotions and a sum score for negative emotions, respectively. M for mean value, SD for standard deviation or n for sample size and % for frequencies were reported to descriptively present the results. For mean value comparisons for the two situations in which interaction with the robot was shown (service situation, care situation), and gender comparison t-tests were calculated. For emotions and attitudes, a one-way ANOVA was calculated in each case, to compare the levels of positive and negative emotions and attitudes (as measured by the questionnaire) for the four appearances of the robot (machine-like, mechanical-human-like, human-like, android).

Multiple linear regressions were run to predict emotions and attitudes respectively. Predictors were dummy coded with situation (service versus care), appearance of the robot (machine-/mechanical-like versus human-like/android), and gender (male versus female). All variables are forced into the linear regression model (method: enter) to investigate their independent contribution. The goodness of fit of the overall model according to Cohen [18] is reported. It was checked for multicollinearity problem in the model as VIF for all variables should be <10, and for auto-correlation problem in the data as the Durbin-Watson-Test should be between the two critical values of $1.5 < d < 2.5$ [34].

3 Results

3.1 Emotions

Emotions Toward Robots. For each situation (S1, S2) and each appearance of the robot (A1, A2, A3, A4) the participants reported their agreement (yes or no) to 30 positive emotions and 30 negative emotions. Taken situations and appearances together, the mean value of the sum score for positive emotions was M = 12.72 (SD = 9.70). The mean value of the sum score for negative emotions was M = 10.31 (SD = 9.84).

When comparing men and women, men (M = 15.15, SD = 9.70) reported on average a higher mean value of the sum score for positive emotions than women (M = 10.72, SD = 9.25). This difference was significant t(529.19) = 5.50, p < .001. Women had a higher mean value of the sum score for negative emotions (M = 12.24, SD = 9.99) than men (M = 7.97, SD = 9.15). This difference was significant t(553.84) = −5.27, p < .001.

On the individual level of the emotion items the participants agreed most frequently with the positive emotions "awake" (75.9%), "attentive" (74.8%) and "interested" (71.9%). The three negative emotions the participants agreed the most were "tense" (49.4%), "unwell" (46.2%) and "dissatisfied" (45.0%).

Emotions Toward Robots in Different Situations. Analyzing the two different situations (S1, S2) separately, the mean value of the sum score for positive emotions was higher in the service situation S1 (M = 14.82, SD = 9.72) than in the care situation S2 (M = 10.67, SD = 9.25) (Table 5). This difference was significant t(557.18) = 5.19, p < .001. The mean value of the sum score for negative emotions was higher in the care situation S2 (M = 12.25, SD = 9.96) than in the service situation S1 (M = 8.32, SD = 9.33) (Table 6). This difference was significant t(560) = −4.83, p < .001.

Emotions Toward Robots of Different Appearance. The mean value of the sum score for positive emotions increased from machine-like A1 (M = 11.03, SD = 9.43), mechanical-human-like A2 (M = 12.76, SD = 10.20), human-like A3 (M = 12.92, SD = 9.44), to android A4 (M = 14.20, SD = 9.26) appearance of the robot (Table 5, Fig. 3). The mean values of the sum score for positive emotions did not differ significantly between the different appearances (F(3, 558) = 2.56, p = .054). A Bonferroni-adjusted post-hoc test showed a significant difference between the machine-like and the android (p = .037) appearance.

The mean value of the sum score for negative emotions decreased from machine-like (M = 11.77, SD = 10.44), mechanical-human-like (M = 10.35, SD = 9.83), human-like (M = 9.84, SD = 9.66), to android (M = 9.26, SD = 9.34) appearance of the robot (Table 6, Fig. 3). The mean values of the sum score for negative emotions did not differ significantly between the different appearances (F(3, 558) = 1.68, p = .171).

Table 5. Positive emotions for situation and appearance [96].

Robot appearance	Service situation (S1)	Care situation (S2)	Both situations
A1: machine-like	M = 13.80 (SD = 10.22)	M = 08.30 (SD = 07.72)	M = 11.03 (SD = 09.43)
A2: mechanical-human-like	M = 15.23 (SD = 10.68)	M = 10.29 (SD = 09.13)	M = 12.76 (SD = 10.20)
A3: human-like	M = 15.77 (SD = 08.86)	M = 10.19 (SD = 09.24)	M = 12.92 (SD = 09.44)
A4: android	M = 14.51 (SD = 09.08)	M = 13.90 (SD = 10.03)	M = 14.20 (SD = 09.55)
Total A1-A4	M = 14.82 (SD = 09.72)	M = 10.67 (SD = 09.25)	M = 12.72 (SD = 09.70)

M: mean value, SD: standard deviation.

Table 6. Negative emotions for situation and appearance [96].

Robot appearance	Service situation (S1)	Care situation (S2)	Both situations
A1: machine-like	M = 08.96 (SD = 09.72)	M = 14.55 (SD = 10.45)	M = 11.77 (SD = 10.44)
A2: mechanical-human-like	M = 07.91 (SD = 09.22)	M = 12.79 (SD = 09.87)	M = 10.35 (SD = 09.83)
A3: human-like	M = 07.71 (SD = 08.81)	M = 11.89 (SD = 10.05)	M = 09.84 (SD = 09.66)
A4: android	M = 09.71 (SD = 09.68)	M = 09.80 (SD = 09.04)	M = 09.26 (SD = 09.34)
Total A1-A4	M = 08.32 (SD = 09.33)	M = 12.25 (SD = 09.96)	M = 10.31 (SD = 09.84)

M: mean value, SD: standard deviation.

Influence of Situation and Appearance on Emotions. In multiple linear regression analysis, situation, appearance of robot, and gender were able to statistically significantly predict the level of positive emotions, F(3, 558) = 22.15, p = .000. The model has no auto-correlation as the value of the Durbin-Watson statistic is 1.716. The R^2 for the overall model was .106 (adjusted R^2 = .102), indicative of a moderate goodness-of-fit. Women expressed less positive emotions than men, the care situation led to less positive

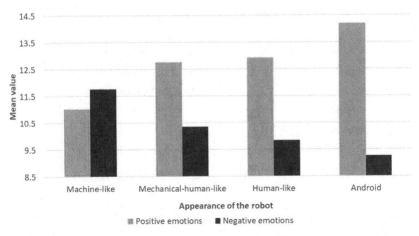

Fig. 3. Mean values of positive and negative emotions for different appearance of the robot.

emotions than the service situation, and the machine-/mechanical-like appearance led to less positive emotions than the human-like/android appearance.

In multiple linear regression analysis, situation and gender were able to statistically significantly predict the level of negative emotions, $F(3, 558) = 19.21$, $p = .000$. The model has no auto-correlation as the value of the Durbin-Watson statistic is 1.88. The R^2 for the overall model was .094 (adjusted $R^2 = .089$), indicative of a weak goodness-of-fit. Women expressed higher negative emotions than men, the care situation led to higher negative emotions than the service situation, no statistically significant influence of appearance on the level of negative emotions could be shown.

3.2 Attitudes

Attitudes Toward Robots. For each situation (S1, S2) and each appearance of the robot (A1, A2, A3, A4) the participants reported their agreement on a five-point scale (1 = do not at all agree to 5 = agree completely) to six items reflecting attitude toward robots (anxiety (ANX1), "afraid to make mistakes"; ANX2, "find robot scary"; attitude toward technology (ATT), "good idea to use the robot"; intention to use (ITU), "I would use the robot"; perceived ease of use (PEOU), "robot is easy to use"; perceived usefulness (PU), "robot is useful" (Table 7).

Table 8 shows the results separated by gender. "Anxiety" and "perceived ease of use" differentiate significantly.

Attitudes Toward Robots in Different Situations. Analyzing the two different situations (S1, S2) separately, the mean value of the items differs significantly for all items except for ANX1 (see Table 9). Indicating a more positive attitude toward robots in the service situation (S1).

Attitudes Toward Robots of Different Appearance. Table 10 shows the mean values and standard deviations of attitudes toward robots for the four different appearances of

Table 7. Attitudes toward robots.

Construct (Code)	Mean (standard deviation)
Anxiety (ANX1)	M = 2.34 (SD = 1.11)
Anxiety (ANX2)	M = 2.61 (SD = 1.30)
Attitude toward technology (ATT)	M = 3.12 (SD = 1.16)
Intention to use (ITU)	M = 3.34 (SD = 1.15)
Perceived ease of use (PEOU)	M = 3.44 (SD = 0.94)
Perceived usefulness (PU)	M = 3.24 (SD = 1.16)

Table 8. Attitudes toward robots by gender.

Construct	Men	Women	T-Test
ANX1	M = 2.08 (SD = 1.00)	M = 2.56 (SD = 1.16)	t(551.39) = −5.33, p < .000*
ANX2	M = 2.37 (SD = 1.25)	M = 2.82 (SD = 1.31)	t(550) = −4.19, p < .000*
ATT	M = 3.22 (SD = 1.14)	M = 3.03 (SD = 1.16)	t(552) = 1.96, p = .051
ITU	M = 3.41 (SD = 1.14)	M = 3.28 (SD = 1.15)	t(551) = 1.32, p = .187
PEOU	M = 3.55 (SD = 0.90)	M = 3.35 (SD = 0.97)	t(551) = 2.48, p = .013*
PU	M = 3.29 (SD = 1.16)	M = 3.21 (SD = 1.16)	t(552) = 0.85, p = .395

M: Mean value, SD: Standard deviation, *: significant

Table 9. Attitude toward robots by situation.

Construct	Service situation (S1)	Care situation (S2)	T-Test
ANX1	M = 2.25 (SD = 1.11)	M = 2.43 (SD = 1.10)	t(552) = −1.93, p = .055
ANX2	M = 2.49 (SD = 1.32)	M = 2.74 (SD = 1.26)	t(550) = −2.26, p = .024*
ATT	M = 3.25 (SD = 1.19)	M = 2.98 (SD = 1.11)	t(548.38) = 2.78, p = .006*
ITU	M = 3.54 (SD = 1.10)	M = 3.14 (Sd = 1.17)	t(551) = 4.13, p < .000*
PEOU	M = 3.61 (SD = 0.91)	M = 3.27 (SD = 0.94)	t(551) = 4.23, p < .000*
PU	M = 3.44 (SD = 1.10)	M = 3.05 (SD = 1.19)	t(552) = 4.06, p < .000*

M: Mean value, SD: Standard deviation, *: significant

the robot. The mean value of ANX1 does not differ significantly between the different appearance of the robot F(3, 550) = 0.38, p = .771. The mean value of ANX2 differs significantly between groups F(3, 548) = 4.61, p = .003. A Bonferroni-adjusted post-hoc test showed a significant difference between the machine-like and the human-like (p = .004) and between the machine-like and the android (p = .022) appearance. ATT does not differ significantly between groups F(3, 550) = 2.40, p = .067. ITU differs significantly between groups F(3, 549) = 3.70, p = .012. A Bonferroni-adjusted post-hoc test showed a significant difference between the machine-like and the human-like (p = .031) appearance. PEOU does not differ significantly between groups F(3, 549) = 0.07, p = .976. PU does not differ significantly between groups F(3, 550) = 1.87, p = .133.

Table 10. Attitude toward robots by appearance.

Construct	Machine-like (A1)	Mechanical-human-like (A2)	Human-like (A3)	Android (A4)
ANX1	M = 2.43 (SD = 1.15)	M = 2.32 (SD = 1.12)	M = 2.30 (SD = 1.06)	M = 2.32 (SD = 1.13)
ANX2	M = 2.94 (SD = 1.32)	M = 2.62 (SD = 1.29)	M = 2.40 (SD = 1.21)	M = 2.49 (SD = 1.32)
ATT	M = 3.00 (SD = 1.13)	M = 2.99 (SD = 1.13)	M = 3.30 (SD = 1.22)	M = 3.19 (SD = 1.13)
ITU	M = 3.15 (SD = 1.19)	M = 3.22 (SD = 1.14)	M = 3.53 (SD = 1.09)	M = 3.46 (SD = 1.14)
PEOU	M = 3.44 (SD = 0.96)	M = 3.44 (SD = 0.95)	M = 3.46 (SD = 0.92)	M = 3.41 (SD = 0.95)
PU	M = 3.12 (SD = 1.17)	M = 3.14 (SD = 1.16)	M = 3.37 (SD = 1.15)	M = 3.35 (SD = 1.15)

M: Mean value, SD: Standard deviation

Influence of Situation and Appearance on Intention to Use the Robot. In multiple linear regression analysis, situation and appearance were able to statistically significantly predict the intention to use (ITU), F(3, 549) = 10.13, p = .000. The model has no auto-correlation as the value of the Durbin-Watson statistic is 2.03. The R^2 for the overall model was .052 (adjusted R^2 = .047), indicative of a weak goodness-of-fit. The care situation led to less intention to use the robot than the service situation. The human-like to android appearance of the robot led to more intention to use the robot than the machine-/mechanical-like appearance. No statistically significant influence of gender on the intention to use the robot could be shown.

4 Discussion

The present study examined emotions and attitudes of Swiss older adults toward robots with different appearances in different situations. As people's impression of robots is socially influenced in every country [105], it is important to have data from many different countries. As far as gender is concerned, although more women participated (54.2%) in the study, this corresponds to the gender distribution in Switzerland from the age group of 65 and over (men: 44.71%, women: 55.29%) [32]. In terms of educational level, however, the sample with a high percentage of well-educated (65.5% tertiary education) does not correspond to the general Swiss population. The distribution of the educational background in Switzerland for older adults (over 65 years) shows more people with secondary education (53%) than with tertiary education (24.2%) [33]. Often, older participants in studies of technology are well educated [e.g. 20,102]. Most participants were interested in technology (71.8% (very) interested in technology) which also is in line with other studies [e.g. 74,101] although Seifert and Schelling [99] found in their study that only

36% of the people 65+ years rather or completely agreed with the statement "I am very interested in new technical things". The proportion of people who had contact with a robot before (24.5%) was slightly lower than in a telephone survey (26%) [38] and in an internet survey in Germany (27%) [82], in the U.S. (43%) and in Japan (31%). But higher than in the Eurobarometer (14%) [28]. A recently published study found in Switzerland 42% of participants had contact with a robot before [64]. The participants lived almost exclusively in private households, which was intended but must be considered when interpreting the results.

The present study found a significant gender effect. Men reporting more positive and women reporting more negative emotions. The gender effect was also significant in the two questions ANX1, ANX2 representing the anxiety construct ("afraid to make a mistake" and "find the robot scary") and the question about perceived ease of use (PEOU). These findings are supported by the review of Broadbent et al. [14] were gender has an impact on how people react to robots, and is in line with the study of Kuo et al. [61] who found in the healthcare sector men having a more positive attitude toward robots than females.

The reported emotions differed significantly in the two different situations. In the service situation (S1, becoming a drink from a robot) more positive emotions and in the care situation (S2, being washed by a robot) more negative emotions were reported. Even five of the six items about attitude toward robots indicate a more positive view of the robot in the service situation (S1). Anxiety was less, positive attitude, intention to use, perceived ease of use and perceived usefulness were higher. There are several possible moderating variables for this effect. The different spatial proximity between the robot and the person in the two different situations could play an important role. Different distances from a robot can influence the level of comfort for the people, and the intermediate distance is rated the best [58]. In the service situation (S1) the robot acts in the intermediate distance and in the care situation (S2) in a close distance. This result corresponds with other studies [e.g. 98].

Differently than expected, the android robot did not evoke more negative emotions than the machine-like, the mechanical-human-like, or the human-like robot. Even if not significantly the mean values of positive emotions increased, and the mean values of negative emotions decreased the more human the appearance of the robot was. Even the mean values of four of the six attitude items toward robot do not differ between the different appearances. Only the anxiety item ANX1 (robot is scary) differs between the machine-like and the human-like and between the machine-like and the android appearance indicating more fear of the machine-like robot. And the intention to use item (ITU) differs significantly between the machine-like and the human-like appearance indicating a lower intention to use the machine-like robot. On one hand, this supports the "uncanny valley" hypothesis indicating a higher acceptance the more human the robot is. But on the other hand, the "valley" with an abrupt drop in acceptance when it is too human-like was not found for the android appearance. A discussion concerning the existence of the "uncanny valley" and its explanations can be found in Broadbendt [13]. In the present study, several possibilities could have affected this result. It could be questionable if the android robot was recognized as a robot. But this explanation can be rejected since it was pointed out in the study instructions and during the study that all images represent robots. Another possible explanation is the recognizable gender of the android robot. The picture shows an android robot that looks like a woman. All other robots cannot be clearly assigned to a gender. Since more women are employed in nursing homes [73], this could have evoked a congruent picture and more positive emotions. In the study of Prakash and Rogers [90], female human-looking faces were partially linked to notions of care or nursing. The independent assessment of the emotions for each vignette can be seen as an advantage of the study but it has to be considered that the participants were not asked which robot they would rather use. In any case, the findings are for example contrary to Arras and Cerqui [5] where only 19% of the participants would prefer a robot with a humanoid appearance, but they are in line with Prakash and Rogers [90] who stated familiarity as the primary reason for a preference of human-looking robots. Tasks that are typically performed by humans can benefit from this circumstance [11]. The findings are in line with Korchut et al. [60] postulating a preference for anthropomorphic appearances. Coming back to the "uncanny valley" it must be considered that in the original formulation of the hypothesis the movement of the robot also has an influence [55]. Overall, participants tended to prefer robots with more human-like appearance and attributes, which can be found in Walters, Syrdal, Dautenhahn, te Boekhorst, and Koay [117] too.

5 Conclusions

The study showed that the specific situation in which a robot interacts with a human has an important influence on positive and negative emotions and on the intention to use the robot. The appearance impacts the intention to use the robot and unpleasant feelings toward the robot. This in turn can influence the acceptance of robots. Additionally, gender also has an effect on emotions and intention to use. Therefore, when developing robots that are designed to interact with older users, it is important to consider the situation in which they will be used, and developers should consider the findings about appearance and gender effects.

Some limitations of the study should be mentioned. As stated above, the study sample is not representative of the general population. Less well-educated or less technology-oriented people should be included in future investigations. It must also be considered that previous experience with robots or prior knowledge about robots leads to a more positive assessment [5]. Since it can be assumed that in the future robotic systems will be increasingly discussed and used in our society, the proportion of people who will already have contact with a robot will increase significantly. A recent Swiss survey already showed a higher proportion of people who already had contact with a robot [64]. In addition, the personal situation of participants should be considered. Persons already in need of care might find the robot conducive to their privacy when helping with personal hygiene. Therefore, in future studies, the characteristics of the sample should be well chosen.

Subsequently, future studies should analyze the specific needs of older adults in real settings. Clearly simulated robot studies and real-world robot studies contribute to knowledge [13] and this simulated study had the advantages of high control over study manipulations, and that it could have been done quickly. The disadvantages were that people were under artificial conditions, therefore the results may not be transferable to real robots and real-world conditions.

This leads to another aspect that should be considered. Because of the study design and the fact that not all robots shown are currently available for testing in Switzerland, the participants only saw pictures of the different robots. Thus, image elements could have influenced the answers, although images were chosen carefully and as similar as possible. But the gap between appearance and movements as described for the "uncanny valley" can be especially great for the android robot. Therefore, robots seen moving in real life might evoke other emotions and attitudes. If technical development and financial considerations make it possible, future studies should be carried out with robots in real life.

Furthermore, many different looking robots exist, but the study used only one example for each category. Future studies should choose more or varying examples, especially if the robot has a gender form, both forms (female and male) must be considered.

Another fact to consider are differences in the videos shown. Both videos showed a woman as the main character but in the service situation (S1) the woman was older, clearly aged over 60 and corresponded more to the study participants what might have affected the responses. Both robots shown in the videos had no heads but could clearly be assigned to a different appearance category. The robot in the service situation (S1) looked machine-like (A1), and the robot in the care situation (S2) mechanical-human-like (A2). The different appearances could have affected the responses too, although the participants were instructed to imagine the robot shown on the picture.

The order of the videos was not varied, all participants first saw the service situation (S1) only the order of the images varied. Therefore, priming effects cannot be excluded. The order of the questions in the questionnaires remained the same too. This might have affected the responses as fatigue effects cannot be ruled out, as the participants had to complete four questionnaires.

Even when other possible target variables for acceptance like trust in robots [70] and not the intention to use can be considered, the present study emphasizes the need to consider the specific situation in which the robot will be used, the congruent appearance of the robot for the specific task and the gender of the end-user when developing robots to support older adults. As there are still unanswered questions, especially arising from the limitations of the present study, further research in this area must follow.

Acknowledgements. Stiftung Suzanne und Hans Biäsch zur Förderung der Angewandten Psychologie funded the project. We thank the foundation for its support and thank the older adults who participated in the study.

References

1. Abbott, R., et al.: How do "robopets" impact the health and well-being of residents in care homes? A systematic review of qualitative and quantitative evidence. Int. J. Older People Nurs. 14(3), e12239 (2019). https://doi.org/10.1111/opn.12239
2. Agnihotri, R., Gaur, S.: Robotics: a new paradigm in geriatric healthcare. Gerontechnology 15(3), 146–161 (2016)

3. Allouch, S.B., van Velsen, L.: Social robots for elderly care: an inventory of promising use cases and business models. Stud. Health Tech. Inf. **270**, 1046–1050 (2020). https://doi.org/10.3233/SHTI200321
4. Arnold, M.B.: Emotion and Personality. Columbia University Press, New York (1960)
5. Arras, K.O., Cerqui, D.: Do we want to share our lives and bodies with robots? A 2000-people survey. Autonomous Systems Lab, Swiss Federal Institute of Technology, EPFL, Lausanne (2005)
6. Atzmüller, C., Steiner, P.M.: Experimental vignette studies in survey research. Methodology **6**, 128–138 (2010). https://doi.org/10.1027/1614-2241/a000014
7. Automation and Control Institute. https://www.acin.tuwien.ac.at/vision-for-robotics/roboter/romeo/. Accessed 01 Jan 2019
8. Baisch, S., et al.: Zeitschrift für Gerontologie und Geriatrie **51**(1), 16–24 (2017). https://doi.org/10.1007/s00391-017-1346-8
9. Barata, A.N.: Social robots as a complementary therapy in chronic, progressive diseases. In: Sequeira, J.S. (ed.) Robotics in Healthcare. AEMB, vol. 1170, pp. 95–102. Springer, Cham (2019). https://doi.org/10.1007/978-3-030-24230-5_5
10. Bemelmans, R., Gelderblom, G.J., Jonker, P., de Witte, L.: Socially assistive robots in elderly care: a systematic review into effects and effectiveness. J. Am. Med. Directors Assoc. **13**(2), 114-120.e1 (2012). https://doi.org/10.1016/j.jamda.2010.10.002
11. Blow, M., Dautenhahn, K., Appleby, A., Nehaniv, C.L., Lee, D.: The art of designing robot faces – dimensions for human-robot interaction. In: Proceedings of the 1st ACM SIGCHI/SIGART Conference on Human–Robot Interaction, pp. 331–332. Association for Computing Machinery, New York (2006). https://doi.org/10.1145/1121241.1121301
12. Breyer, B., Bluemke, M.: Deutsche Version der Positive and Negative Affect Schedule PANAS (GESIS Panel). Zusammenstellung sozialwissenschaftlicher Items und Skalen (2016). https://doi.org/10.6102/zis242
13. Broadbent, E.: Interactions with robots: the truths we reveal about ourselves. Annu. Rev. Psychol. **68**(1), 627–652 (2017). https://doi.org/10.1146/annurev-psych-010416-043958
14. Broadbent, E., Stafford, R., MacDonald, B.: Acceptance of healthcare robots for the older population: review and future directions. Int. J. Soc. Robot. **1**, 319 (2009). https://doi.org/10.1007/s12369-009-0030-6
15. Broadbent, E., Tamagawa, R., Kerse, N., Knock, B., Patience, A., MacDonald, B.: Retirement home staff and residents' preferences for healthcare robots. In: The 18th IEEE International Symposium on Robot and Human Interactive Communication, Toyama, pp. 645–650. IEEE (2009)
16. Broekens, J., Heerink, M., Rosendal, H.: Assistive social robots in elderly care: a review. Gerontechnology **8**(2), 94–103 (2009). https://doi.org/10.4017/gt.2009.08.02.002.00
17. Chita-Tegmark, M., Ackerman, J.M., Scheutz, M.: Effects of assistive robot behavior on impressions of patient psychological attributes: vignette-based human-robot interaction study. J. Med. Internet Res. **21**(6), e13729 (2019). https://doi.org/10.2196/13729
18. Cohen, J.: Statistical Power Analysis for the Behavioral Sciences, 2nd edn. L. Erlbaum Associates, Hillsdale (1988)
19. Compagna, D., Marquardt, M.: Zur Evaluation von Mensch-Roboter Interaktionen (MRI) – ein methodischer Beitrag aus soziologischer Perspektive. Working Papers kultur- und techniksoziologische Studien 3, p. 18. Universität Duisburg-Essen, Duisburg (2015)
20. Dahms, R., Haesner, M.: Prävention und Gesundheitsförderung **13**(1), 46–52 (2017). https://doi.org/10.1007/s11553-017-0610-5
21. Davis, F.D., Bagozzi, R.P., Warshaw, P.R.: User acceptance of computer technology: a comparison of two theoretical models. Manage. Sci. **35**(8), 982–1003 (1989)

22. Decker, M.: Ein Abbild des Menschen: Humanoide Roboter. In: Bölker, M., Gutmann, M., Hesse, W. (eds.) Information und Menschenbild, pp. 41–62. Springer, Heidelberg (2010). https://doi.org/10.1007/978-3-642-04742-8_3

23. De Graaf, M., Allouch, S.M.: Exploring influencing variables for the acceptance of social robots. Robot. Autonom. Syst. **61**(12), 1476–1486 (2013). https://doi.org/10.1016/j.robot.2013.07.007

24. DiSalvo, C.F., Gemperle, F., Forlizzi, J., Kiesler, S.: All robots are not created equal: the design and perception of humanoid robot heads. In: Proceedings of the 4th Conference on Designing Interactive Systems: Process, Practices, Methods, and Techniques, London, pp. 321–326. ACM (2002)

25. Ebert, D.D., Christ, O., Berking, M.: Entwicklung und Validierung eines Fragebogens zur emotionsspezifischen Selbsteinschätzung emotionaler Kompetenzen (SEK-ES). Diagnostica **59**(1), 17–32 (2013). https://doi.org/10.1026/0012-1924/a000079

26. Eftring, H., Frennert, S.: Zeitschrift für Gerontologie und Geriatrie **49**(4), 274–281 (2016). https://doi.org/10.1007/s00391-016-1064-7

27. Ekman, P., Friesen, W.V., Ellsworth, P.: What emotion categories or dimensions can observers judge from facial behavior? In: Ekman, P. (ed.) Emotion in the Human Face, pp. 39–55. Cambridge University Press, New York (1982)

28. European Commission: Special Eurobarometer 460. Attitudes towards the impact of digitisation and automation on daily life (2017). https://ec.europa.eu/jrc/communities/sites/jrccties/files/ebs_460_en.pdf

29. Eurostat.: Bevölkerungsstruktur und Bevölkerungsalterung (2019). https://ec.europa.eu/eurostat/statistics-explained/index.php?title=Population_structure_and_ageing/de#Der_Anteil_.C3.A4lterer_Menschen_nimmt_weiter_zu. Accessed 10 Aug 2020

30. F&P PersonalRobotics. https://www.fp-robotics.com/de/service-robotics/. Accessed 21 Jan 2019

31. Fan, L., Scheutz, M., Lohani, M., McCoy, M., Stokes, C.: Do we need emotionally intelligent artificial agents? First results of human perceptions of emotional intelligence in humans compared to robots. In: Beskow, J., Peters, C., Castellano, G., O'Sullivan, C., Leite, I., Kopp, S. (eds.) Intelligent Virtual Agents. Springer, Cham (2017). https://doi.org/10.1007/978-3-319-67401-8_15

32. Federal Statistical Office: Ständige Wohnbevölkerung nach Alter, Geschlecht und Staatsangehörigkeitskategorie, 2010–2019 (2020). https://www.bfs.admin.ch/bfs/de/home/statistiken/bevoelkerung/stand-entwicklung/alter-zivilstand-staatsangehoerigkeit.assetdetail.13707177.html

33. Federal Statistical Office: Bildungsstand (2020). https://www.bfs.admin.ch/bfs/de/home/statistiken/wirtschaftliche-soziale-situation-bevoelkerung/gleichstellung-frau-mann/bildung/bildungsstand.html

34. Field, A.: Discovering Statistics Using SPSS, (and Sex and Drugs and Rock 'n' Roll), 3rd edn. SAGE, London (2009)

35. Flandorfer, P.: Population ageing and socially assistive robots for elderly persons: the importance of sociodemographic factors for user acceptance. Int. J. Population Res. 829835 (2012). https://doi.org/10.1155/2012/829835

36. Fraunhofer-Institut für Produktionstechnik und Automatisierung Homepage, https://www.care-o-bot.de/de/care-o-bot-3/download/videos.html. Accessed 10 Aug 2020

37. Frijda, N.H.: The Emotions. Cambridge University Press, New York (1986)

38. Forsa. Politik- und Sozialforschung GmbH: "Service-Robotik: Mensch-Technik-Interaktion im Alltag". Ergebnisse einer repräsentativen Befragung. Berlin (2016). https://www.bmbf.de/files/BMBF_forsa_Robotik_FINAL2016.pdf

39. Gaul, S., et al.: Technikakzeptanz als integraler Bestandteil der Entwicklung medizintechnischer Produkte. In: Ambient Assisted Living 2010: 3. Deutscher AAL-Kongress mit Ausstellung, Assistenzsysteme im Dienste des Menschen – zuhause und unterwegs, Tagungsbeitrag. Berlin (2010)

40. Georgia Tech: Healthcare Robotics Lab. https://sites.gatech.edu/hrl/robotic-nurse-assistant/. Accessed 10 Aug 2020

41. Goher, K.M., Mansouri, N., Fadlallah, S.O.: Assessment of personal care and medical robots from older adults' perspective. Robot. Biomimetics 4(1), 1–7 (2017). https://doi.org/10.1186/s40638-017-0061-7

42. Graf, B., Heyer, T., Klein, B., Wallhoff, F.: Servicerobotik für den demografischen Wandel. Mögliche Einsatzfelder und aktueller Entwicklungsstand [Service robots in elderly care. Possible application areas and current state of developments]. Bundesgesundheitsblatt Gesundheitsforschung Gesundheitsschutz 56(8), 1145–1152 (2013). https://doi.org/10.1007/s00103-013-1755-9

43. Gray, J.A.: The Neuropsychology of Anxiety. Oxford University Press, Oxford (1982)

44. Grimm, J.: State-Trait-Anxiety Inventory nach Spielberger. Deutsche Lang- und Kurzversion. Methodenforum der Universität Wien: MF-Working Paper 2009/02 (2009)

45. Hawley-Hague, H., Boulton, E., Hall, A., Pfeiffer, K., Todd, C.: Older adults' perceptions of technologies aimed at falls prevention, detection or monitoring: a systematic review. Int. J. Med. Informatics 83(6), 416–426 (2014). https://doi.org/10.1016/j.ijmedinf.2014.03.002

46. Heerink, M., Kröse, B., Evers, V., Wielinga, B.: Assessing acceptance of assistive social agent technology by older adults: the Almere model. Int. J. Soc. Robot. 2, 361–375 (2010). https://doi.org/10.1007/s12369-010-0068-5

47. Ho, C.-C., MacDorman, K.F.: Measuring the uncanny valley effect. Int. J. Soc. Robot. 9(1), 129–139 (2016). https://doi.org/10.1007/s12369-016-0380-9

48. Hung, L., et al.: The benefits of and barriers to using a social robot PARO in care settings: a scoping review. BMC Geriatr. 19(1), 232 (2019). https://doi.org/10.1186/s12877-019-1244-6

49. Hwang, J., Park, T., Hwang, W.: The effects of overall robot shape on the emotions invoked in users and the perceived personalities of robot. Appl. Ergon. 44, 459–471 (2013). https://doi.org/10.1016/j.apergo.2012.10.010

50. Izard, C.E.: The Face of Emotion. Appleton-Century-Crofts, New York (1971)

51. James, W.: What is an emotion? Mind 9(34), 188–205 (1884)

52. Janke, W., Debus, G.: Die Eigenschafswörterliste: EWL; eine mehrdimensionale Methode zur Beschreibung von Aspekten des Befindens. Hogrefe Verlag für Psychologie, Göttingen (1978)

53. Janowski, K., Ritschel, H., Lugrin, B., André, E.: Sozial interagierende Roboter in der Pflege. In: Bendel, O. (ed.) Pflegeroboter, pp. 63–87. Springer, Wiesbaden (2018). https://doi.org/10.1007/978-3-658-22698-5_4

54. Jost, C., et al.: Human-Robot Interaction Evaluation methods and their standardization. Springer, Cham (2020). https://doi.org/10.1007/978-3-030-42307-0

55. Kätsyri, J., Förger, K., Mäkäräinen, M., Takala, T.: A review of empirical evidence on different uncanny valley hypotheses: support for perceptual mismatch as one road to the valley of eeriness. Front. Psychol. 6, 390 (2015)

56. Kessler, J., Schroeter, C., Gross, H.-M.: Approaching a person in a socially acceptable manner using a fast marching planner. In: Jeschke, S., Liu, H., Schilberg, D. (eds.) ICIRA 2011. LNCS (LNAI), vol. 7102, pp. 368–377. Springer, Heidelberg (2011). https://doi.org/10.1007/978-3-642-25489-5_36

57. Kiesler, S., Hinds, P.: Introduction to this special issue on human-robot interaction. Human-Comput. Interact. 19, 1–8 (2004)

58. Koay, K.L., Dautenhahn, K., Woods, S., Walters, M.L.: Empirical results from using a comfort level device in human-robot interaction studies. In: Proceedings of the 1st ACM SIGCHI/SIGART Conference on Human-Robot Interaction, pp. 194–201 (2006)
59. Khosla, R., Nguyen, K., Chu, M.-T.: Human robot engagement and acceptability in residential aged care. Int. J. Hum. Comput. Interact. **33**, 510–522 (2017). https://doi.org/10.1080/10447318.2016.1275435
60. Korchut, A., et al.: Challenges for service robots – requirements of elderly adults with cognitive impairments. Front. Neurol. **8**, 228 (2017)
61. Kuo, I.H., et al.: Age and gender factors in user accceptance of healthcare robots. In: The 18th IEEE International Symposium on Robots and Human Interactive Communication, Toyama (2009)
62. Lang, G.: Zur Befragung und Befragbarkeit von kognitiv eingeschränkten und demenziell veränderten Menschen in Altern- und Pflegeheimen. In: Amann, A., Kolland, F. (eds.) Das erzwungene Paradies des Alters? Weitere Fragen an eine Kritische Gerontologie, pp. 207–215. Springer VS, Wiesbaden (2014)
63. Lauckner, M., Kobiela, F., Manzey, D.: 'Hey robot, please step back!' - Exploration of a spatial threshold of comfort for human-mechanoid spatial interaction in a hallway scenario. In: The 23rd IEEE International Symposium on Robot and Human Interactive Communication, Edinburgh, pp. 780–787 (2014). https://doi.org/10.1109/ROMAN.2014.6926348
64. Lehmann, S., Ruf, E., Misoch, S.: Robot use for older adults – attitudes, wishes and concerns. First results from Switzerland. In: Stephanidis, C., Antona, M. (eds.) HCII 2020. CCIS, vol. 1226, pp. 64–70. Springer, Cham (2020). https://doi.org/10.1007/978-3-030-50732-9_9
65. Maalouf, N., Sidaoui, A., Elhajj, I.H., Asmar, D.: Robotics in nursing: a scoping review. J. Nurs. Scholarsh. Official Publ. Sigma Theta Tau Int. Honor Soc. Nurs. **50**(6), 590–600 (2018). https://doi.org/10.1111/jnu.12424
66. MacDorman, K.F., Chattopadhyay, D.: Reducing consistency in human realism increases the uncanny valley effect; increasing category uncertainty does not. Cognition **146**, 190–205 (2016). https://doi.org/10.1016/j.cognition.2015.09.019
67. MacDorman, K.F., Ishiguro, H.: The uncanny advantage of using androids in cognitive and social science research. Interact. Stud. **7**, 297–337 (2006)
68. Mara, M., Appel, M.: Roboter im Gruselgraben: Warum uns menschenähnliche Maschinen oft unheimlich sind. In-Mind Magazin 5. Medienpsychologie Teil 2: Medien, Nachrichten und wir (2015)
69. Marek, K.D., Rantz, M.J.: Ageing in place: a new model for long-term care. Nurs. Adm. Q. **24**(3), 1–1 (2000)
70. Mathur, M.B., Reichling, D.B.: Navigating a social world with robot partners: a quantitative cartography of the uncanny valley. Cognition **146**, 22–32 (2016). https://doi.org/10.1016/j.cognition.2015.09.008
71. McDougall, W.: An Introduction to Social Psychology. Luce, Boston (1926)
72. McGlynn, S.A., Kemple, S., Mitzner, T.L., King, C.A., Rogers, W.A.: Understanding the potential of PARO for healthy older adults. Int. J. Hum Comput Stud. **100**, 33–47 (2017). https://doi.org/10.1016/j.ijhcs.2016.12.004
73. Mercay, C., Grünig, A.: Gesundheitspersonal in der Schweiz – Zukünftiger Bedarf bis 2030 und die Folgen für den Nachwuchsbedarf (Obsan Bulletin 12/2016). Schweizerisches Gesundheitsobservatorium, Neuchâtel (2016)
74. Mies, C.: Akzeptanz von Smart Home Technologien: Einfluss von subjektivem Pflegebedarf und Technikerfahrung bei älteren Menschen. Untersuchung im Rahmen des Projekts «Accepting Smart Homes». Diplomarbeit., Wien (2011)
75. Miklósi, Á., Korondi, P., Matellán, V., Gácsi, M.: Ethorobotics: a new approach to human-robot relationship. Front. Psychol. **8**, 958 (2017). https://doi.org/10.3389/fpsyg.2017.00958

76. Miraikan, National Museum of Emerging Science and Innovation. https://www.mir aikan.jst.go.jp/en/online/communication/profile/otonaroid.html?width=560&height=1534. Accessed 28 Jan 2019

77. Misoch, S., Pauli, C., Ruf, E.: Technikakzeptanzmodelle: Theorieübersicht und kritische Würdigung mit Fokus auf ältere Nutzer/innen (60+). In: Weidner, R. (ed.) Technische Unterstützungssysteme, die die Menschen wirklich wollen, pp. 107–115. Konferenzband, Hamburg (2016)

78. Mollenkopf, H., Kaspar, R.: Technisierte Umwelten als Handlungs- und Erlebensräume älterer Menschen. In: Backes, G.M., Clemens, W., Künemund, H. (eds.) Lebensformen und Lebensführung im Alter, pp. 193–221. VS Verlag für Sozialwissenschaften, Wiesbaden (2004)

79. Monathan, J.L.: I don't know it but I like you – the influence of non-conscious affect on person perception. Hum. Commun. Res. 24(4), 480–500 (1998). https://doi.org/10.1111/j. 1468-2958.1998.tb00428.x

80. Mori, M.: The uncanny valley. Energy 7, 33–35 (1970)

81. Mowrer, O.H.: Learning Theory and Behaviour. Wiley, New York (1960)

82. Nitto, H., Taniyama, D., Inagaki, H.: Social acceptance and impact of robots and artificial intelligence. Findings of survey in Japan, the US and Germany. Nomura Research Institute (NRI Papers, 211) (2017). https://www.nri.com/-/media/Corporate/en/Files/PDF/knowle dge/report/cc/papers/2017/np2017211.pdf?la=en&hash=A730998FD55F6D58DF95F347 9E3B709FC8EF83F4

83. Nomura, T., Kanda, T., Suzuki, T., Kato, K.: Experimental investigation into influence of negative attitudes toward robots on human-robot interaction. AI Soc. 20(2), 138–150 (2006). https://doi.org/10.1007/s00146-005-0012-7

84. Nomura, T., Kanda, T., Suzuki, T., Kato, K.: Prediction of human behavior in human-robot interaction using psychological scales for anxiety and negative attitudes toward robots. IEEE Trans. Rob. 24(2), 442–451 (2008)

85. Oatley, K., Johnson-Laird, P.N.: Towards a cognitive theory of emotions. Cogn. Emot. 1, 29–50 (1987)

86. Ortony, A., Turner, T.J.: What's basic about basic emotions? Psychol. Rev. 97(3), 315–331 (1990)

87. Panksepp, J.: Toward a general psychobiological theory of emotions. Behav. Brain Sci. 5, 407–467 (1982)

88. Parviainen, J., Turja, T., Van Aerschot, L.: Robots and human touch in care: desirable and non-desirable robot assistance. In: Ge, S.S., Cabibihan, J.-J., Salichs, M.A., Broadbent, E., He, H., Wagner, A.R., Castro-González, Á. (eds.) ICSR 2018. LNCS (LNAI), vol. 11357, pp. 533–540. Springer, Cham (2018). https://doi.org/10.1007/978-3-030-05204-1_52

89. Plutchik, R.: A general psychoevolutionary theory of emotion. In: Plutchik, R., Kellerman, H. (eds.) Emotion: Theory, Research, and Experience, Theories of Emotion, vol. 1., p. 31. Academic Press, New York (1980)

90. Prakash, A., Rogers, W.A.: Why some humanoid faces are perceived more positively than others: effects of human-likeness and task. Int. J. Soc. Robot. 7(2), 309–331 (2014). https:// doi.org/10.1007/s12369-014-0269-4

91. Pu, L., Moyle, W., Jones, C., Todorovic, M.: The effectiveness of social robots for older adults: a systematic review and meta-analysis of randomized controlled studies. Gerontologist 59(1), e37–e51 (2019). https://doi.org/10.1093/geront/gny046

92. Ray, C., Mondada, F., Siegwart, R.: What do people expect from robots? In: Proceedings of the IEEE/RSJ International Conference on Intelligent Robots and Systems, pp. 3816–3821. Nice (2008)

93. Robinson, H., MacDonald, B., Broadbent, E.: The role of healthcare robots for older people at home: a review. Int. J. Soc. Robot. **6**(4), 575–591 (2014). https://doi.org/10.1007/s12369-014-0242-2

94. Rosenthal-von der Pütten, A.M., Krämer, N.C., Hoffmann, L., Sobieraj, S., Eimler, S.C.: An experimental study on emotional reactions towards a robot. Int. J. Soc. Robot. **5**(1), 17–34 (2013)

95. Rosenthal-von der Pütten, A.M., et al.: Investigations on empathy towards humans and robots using fMRI. Comput. Hum. Behav. **33**, 201–212 (2014)

96. Ruf, E., Lehmann, S., Misoch, S.: Service robots: emotions of older adults in different situations. In: Guldemond, N., Ziefle, M., Maciaszek, L. (eds.) Proceedings of the 6th Internactional Conference on Information and Communication Technologies for Ageing Well and e-Health, pp. 15–25 (2020). https://doi.org/10.5220/0009324500150025

97. Scopelliti, M., Giuliani, M.V., Fornara, F.: Robots in a domestic setting: a psychological approach. Univ. Access Inf. Soc. **4**, 146–155 (2005)

98. Seibt, J., Nørskov, M., Schack Andersen, S.: What Social Robots Can and Should Do. Proceedings of Robophilosophy/TRANSOR. IOS Press, Amsterdam (2016)

99. Seifert, A., Schelling, H.R.: Digitale Senioren. Nutzung von Informations- und Kommunikationstechnologien (IKT) durch Menschen ab 65 Jahren in der Schweiz im Jahr 2015. Pro Senectute Verlag, Zürich (2015)

100. Sixsmith, A., Gutmann, G.M.: Technologies for Active Aging, vol. 9. Springer, New York (2013). https://doi.org/10.1007/978-1-4419-8348-0

101. Stadelhofer, C.: Möglichkeiten und Chancen der Internetnutzung durch Ältere. Zeitschrift für Gerontologie und Geriatrie **33**, 186–194 (2000)

102. Steinert, A., Haesner, M., Tetley, A., Steinhagen-Thiessen, E.: Prävention und Gesundheitsförderung **10**(4), 281–286 (2015). https://doi.org/10.1007/s11553-015-0510-5

103. Steyer, R., Schwenkmezger, P., Notz, P., Eid, M.: Der Mehrdimensionale Befindlichkeitsfragebogen (MDBF) Handanweisung. Hogrefe, Göttingen (1997)

104. Strait, M.K., et al.: Understanding the uncanny: both atypical features and category ambiguity provoke aversion toward humanlike robots. Front. Psychol. **8**, 1366 (2017)

105. Suwa, S., et al.: Exploring perceptions toward home-care robots for older people in Finland, Ireland, and Japan: a comparative questionnaire study. Arch. Gerontol. Geriatr. **91**, 104178 (2020). https://doi.org/10.1016/J.archger.2020.104178

106. TelepresenceRobots. https://telepresencerobots.com/robosoft's-kompai. Accessd 28 Jan 2019

107. Tomkins, S.S.: Affect theory. In: Scherer, K.R., Ekman, P. (eds.) Approaches to Emotion, pp. 163–195. Erlbaum, Hillsdale (1984)

108. Torta, E., et al.: Evaluation of a small socially-assistive humanoid robot in intelligent homes for the care of the elderly. J. Intell. Rob. Syst. **76**(1), 57–71 (2014). https://doi.org/10.1007/s10846-013-0019-0

109. Vaupel, J.: Setting the stage: a generation of centenarians? Washington Q. **23**(3), 197–200 (2000)

110. Venkatesh, V., Bala, H.: Technology acceptance model 3 and a research agenda on interventions. Decis. Sci. **39**, 273–315 (2008). https://doi.org/10.1111/j.1540-5915.2008.00192.x

111. Venkatesh, V., Davis, F.D.: A theoretical extension of the technology acceptance model: four longitudinal field studies. Manage. Sci. **46**, 186–204 (2000). https://doi.org/10.1287/mnsc.46.2.186.11926

112. Venkatesh, V., Morris, M.G., Davis, G.B., Davis, F.D.: User acceptance of information technology: Toward a unified view. Manage. Inf. Syst. Q. **27**(3), 425–478 (2003)

113. Von Zerssen, D., Petermann, F.: Befindlichkeits-Skala. Revidierte Fassung (Bf-SR). Hogrefe (2011).

114. Wachsmuth, I.: Robots like me: challenges and ethical issues in aged care. Front. Psychol. **9**, 432 (2018). https://doi.org/10.3389/fpsyg.2018.00432
115. Walters, M.L, Dautenhahn K., Te Boekhorst, R., Koay, K.L., Syrdal, D.S., Nehaniv, C.L.: An empirical framework for human-robot proxemics. In: Proceedings of the New Frontiers in Human-Robot Interaction (2009)
116. Walters, M.L., Koay, K.L., Syrdal, D.S., Dautenhahn, K., Te Boekhorst, R.: Preferences and perceptions of robot appearance and embodiment in human-robot interaction trials. In: Proceedings of New Frontiers in Human-Robot Interaction (2009)
117. Walters, M.L., Syrdal, D.S., Dautenhahn, K., te Boekhorst, R., Koay, K.L.: Avoiding the uncanny valley: robot appearance, personality and consistency of behavior in an attention-seeking home scenario for a robot companion. Auton. Robots **24**(2), 159–178 (2008). https://doi.org/10.1007/s10514-007-9058-3
118. Watson, J.B.: Behaviorism. University of Chicago Press, Chicago (1930)
119. Weiner, B., Graham, S.: An attributional approach to emotional development. In: Izard, C.E., Kagan, J., Zajonc, R.B. (eds.) Emotions, Cognition, and Behavior, pp. 167–191. Cambridge University Press, New York (1984)
120. Wirtz, J., et al.: Brave new world: service robots in the frontline. J. Serv. Manage. **29**, 907–931 (2018). https://doi.org/10.1108/JOSM-04-201-0119
121. World Health Organization: World report on ageing and health. World Health Organization, Geneva (2015)
122. World Health Organization: Global priority research agenda for improving access to high-quality affordable assistive technology. World Health Organization, Geneva (2017). https://apps.who.int/iris/bitstream/10665/254660/1/WHO-EMP-IAU-2017.02-eng.pdf
123. Wu, Y.H., Fassert, C., Rigaud, A.S.: Designing robots for the elderly: appearance issue and beyond. Arch. Gerontol. Geriatr. **54**(1), 121–126 (2012). https://doi.org/10.1016/j.archger.2011.02.003
124. Wu, Y.-H., Wrobel, J., Cornuet, M., Kerhervé, H., Damnée, S., Rigaud, A.-S.: Acceptance of an assistive robot in older adults: a mixed-method study of human-robot interaction over a 1-month period in the living lab setting. Clin. Interv. Aging **9**, 801–811 (2014). https://doi.org/10.2147/CIA.S56435

IoT Environment for Monitoring Human Movements: Hip Fracture Rehabilitation Case

Akash Gupta$^{(\boxtimes)}$, Khalid Al-Naime, and Adnan Al-Anbuky

School of Engineering, Computer and Mathematical Sciences,
Auckland University of Technology, Auckland, New Zealand
`{akash.gupta,khalid.alnaime,adnan.anbuky}@aut.ac.nz`

Abstract. Hip fracture incidence increases with age and possess a serious long-term devastating impact on the physical functionality of the older population and on their ability to live independently. Increased risk in mortality rate, movement restriction, person's well-being and loss of independence are some of the significant problems associated with the injury. Rehabilitation plays a significant role in recovery of the muscle strength, boosting the quality of life and improving the physical functionality in all stages of care. The rehabilitation program has activity movements relevant to an injury that needs to be performed under pre-defined supervised or unsupervised environment. Continual monitoring of these activity movements in any environment can significantly help in follow up the correct implementation of a rehabilitation program. The ever-growing technology like Internet of Things (IoT) and advancements in digital health revolutionizing all industries and markets could be leveraged upon in advancing and converting the conventional rehabilitation care into a smart rehabilitation care. This paper proposes an IoT environment for long-term monitoring of hip fracture rehabilitation related activity movements. Functionality of the attributes involved in the environment have been discussed pragmatically through experimental analysis. Results reflect that the environment can offer flexibility for different movement monitoring, analysis and visualisation applications.

Keyword: Rehabilitation · Activity movement monitoring · Internet of Things (IoT) · Hip fracture · Remote Monitoring

1 Introduction

According to World Health Organisation (WHO), it has been projected that the world's elderly population aged 65 and above is rapidly growing and is expected to increase from 900 million in 2015 to 2 billion by 2050 [1]. Hip fracture is common event among older population and a critical life-threatening injury. Rehabilitation plays a guaranteeing role in recovery and enhancing the quality of life of a person suffering from such type of injury. It is an essential part of healthcare especially considering the continual rising ageing population, associated prevalence of chronic disability and deterioration of physical functionality due to illness or injury [2]. An 18% increase in the incidence of non-communicable diseases like stroke, hip fracture and cancer has been observed in the last

© Springer Nature Switzerland AG 2021
M. Ziefle et al. (Eds.): ICT4AWE 2020, CCIS 1387, pp. 44–63, 2021.
https://doi.org/10.1007/978-3-030-70807-8_3

10 years [3]. Several rehabilitation programs are available that aids in the recovery and improvement of the physical functionality. However, the efficacy of the program is yet ambiguous as the rehabilitation mostly happens when patient is living in a rest home independently and unsupervised. Therefore, healthcare professionals lack the short-time history and real-time activity movement data of the patients, affecting the necessary and accurate support for the patient to achieve their personalised goals. This renders a critical global challenge to the existing healthcare and medical service system. As a result, it urges for the development of timely monitoring system. This should provide a comprehensive care plan program to each cause, assist healthcare professionals to constantly monitor and recognize patient detail movement activities remotely, examine their improvement levels, whether the activities are done in supervised (in hospital and clinics) or unsupervised (at home and outdoor) environment, have a timely follow up and emergency care [4].

Internet of things (IoT) also known by industrial internet or internet of everything is an ever-growing new technology paradigm revolutionising all industries and markets in essential ways [5, 6]. It provides a comprehensive environment by integrating hardware, large number of heterogeneous physical things, software and thus enabling them to collect, exchange data, interact, and communicate. Integration of IoT with healthcare can significantly help in reduction of the cost, improve quality of life and enrich user experience. However, it still possesses lots of promising challenges like latency, constrained resources, data interoperability, storage and management, security and ubiquitous access. Even though IoT based healthcare system has evolved over the recent years and has the potential to upsurge numerous healthcare applications for instance elderly healthcare rehabilitation, less attention has been given to the remote human movement monitoring of patient's rehabilitation of post-operative hip fracture rehabilitation cases.

This paper proposed an IoT environment for monitoring hip fracture rehabilitation activity movements. The environment lays out the ground for establishing an overall rehabilitation long-term movement monitoring system. The significance, role and responsibilities of each functionality involved within the system design has been discussed through hip fracture rehabilitation activity movement data experimental analysis.

The organisation of the paper is as follows: Next section describes the related work pertaining to activity recognition techniques, IoT system architecture proposed and implemented by the existing literatures within the field of healthcare. Section 3 represents the proposed rehabilitation activity movement monitoring architecture. Section 4 discusses the architectural functionality implementation on hip fracture rehabilitation movement monitoring. Section 5 concludes the paper.

2 Related Work

Due to an unprecedented advancement in IoT, many different prototypes and services has been proposed and established. However, within healthcare system, partial information is available pertaining to the role and contribution of each attribute in establishing an IoT environment for rehabilitation activity movement monitoring system. The devices involved in an IoT architectural system are capable of sensing data acquisition, computation, communication and in the controlling the overall system environment.

Recognition of human activity movements aids in providing the information about person's identity, daily physical changes and psychological state. This further helps in human-to-human interaction and interpersonal relations. For activity movement recognition and monitoring of the overall process, wearable sensing devices plays an important part in acquiring the patient activity movement data. Wireless body worn wearable sensors have gained the most popularity because of the sensor miniaturization using Inertial Measurement Unit (IMU). Among these, triaxial accelerometer is the most widely accepted sensor for monitoring Activities of Daily Living (ADL's), posture, falls and movement classification. Different digital signal processing [7, 8], inclination angle, threshold and statistical based technique has been used by [9–11] to classify both static and ambulatory activities using a single tri-axial accelerometer. Good accuracy level of 97.65% has been achieved in categorizing ADL using accelerometer but the recognition rate reduced drastically while classifying ADL with gesture-based activity movements [12]. This is because most the gesture-based movements are multi-directional and basing the recognition algorithm on axis dependent technique might not be feasible. Moreover, it also restricts the user to wear the sensor in a specific orientation rather than making the algorithm immune to potential errors in aligning the sensors with body or anatomical axis.

Many different healthcare architectures pertaining to healthcare have been proposed [5, 13, 14]. However, none of them has discussed the system operation based on real-life testing of the human on any application. Moreover, limited information is provided on how each level in the IoT environment could contribute to offering a more robust and scalable system. It also lacks in explaining the system implementation challenges and how one could overcome and adjust for satisfying different applications. Considering all these factors and challenges in mind, [15] proposed an IoT based system architecture using a decentralized approach where the involved attributes in the layer could be used for handling computational and decision-making capabilities. This could significantly aid in reducing the data packet size and minimize the communication latency duration. However, this approach has not been employed in real-life healthcare application where the reaction and response time is of great concern. Understanding the significance and distributing the functionality load at each level could be of great interest while laying out the IoT environment for rehabilitation activity movement monitoring. Next section discusses the proposed rehabilitation activity movement architecture.

3   Rehabilitation Activity Movement Monitoring Architecture

The conceptual architecture proposed for monitoring the post-operative hip fracture rehabilitation activity is illustrated in Fig. 1 below.

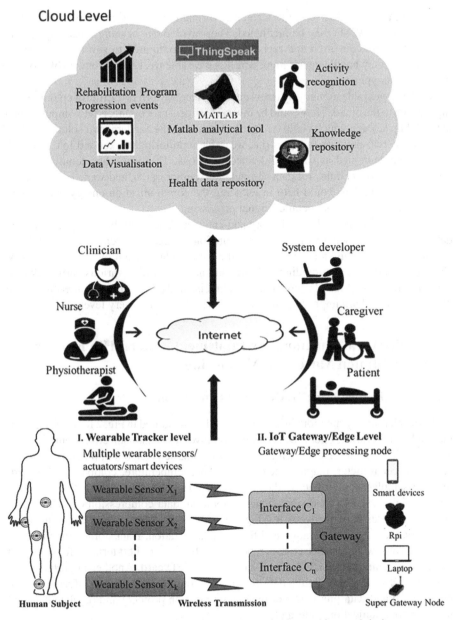

Fig. 1. Rehabilitation activity movement monitoring architectural design.

The architectural design is mainly composed of three level functionalities. These are wearable monitoring tracker level, IoT gateway or edge level, and cloud level functionalities. Each of these levels plays a unique and significant role in the overall rehabilitation movement monitoring process.

The wearable tracker report to a gateway through embedded protocol(s) like Bluetooth, ZigBee or Wi-Fi may be facilitated. They involve one or more sensing types and the rate of data acquisition and reporting could be configured to suit the application. The gateway may handle one or more wireless wearable tracker that may involve one or more sensing types.

Both the wearable monitoring tracker and IoT gateway offers the role of communicating the data to the cloud. They could be involved in local processing, edge computing and data backup storage which could be handled as part of the fundamental solution. Alternatively, the two-network modules (i.e. wearable monitoring tracker and IoT gateway) could be implemented as software defined functions. This could be accomplished by operating the two modules for data computation, compression, and some level of activity classification. This could help in reducing the communication energy expenditure and relieve the cloud from detailed signal processing.

At the cloud level, real time, history and knowledge data will be managed. Involved data processing, activity recognition, rehabilitation progression event detection and data visualization modelling takes place using the data available from the cloud repository. The cloud facilitates in providing key user interaction with the various parties like the patient, caregiver, system developer, nurse, clinician and physiotherapist as each of them play their own role in improving the patient rehabilitation recovery levels.

4   Architectural Functionality Implementation on Hip Fracture Rehabilitation Movement Monitoring

4.1   Wearable Monitoring Tracker Level Functionality

At this level, four key functionalities are involved as illustrated in Fig. 2 for offering modular and configurable system. Data acquisition involves sensor selection, sampling rate and acquisition duration. One or more sensors may be selected out of numerous sensors such as accelerometer, magnetometer, gyroscope, temperature, compass and humidity. The sampled sensed data is then be subjected to the data computation that may involve digital signal processing, signal calibration, data compression etc. Other processing activities may involve managing the analysis and formation of communication messages, the mode of operation and time synchronization. Data storage functionality comprises of raw and processed data repository. This can be short term buffer storage at main memory and long-term back up storage using SD card. Another important functionality is that of managing the data communication protocol. This in effect configure the physical and data link layers of the communication protocol and regulate data and message communication pattern [16].

In monitoring hip-fracture rehabilitation activity movement, a wearable tracker is designed based on Microduino existing modules. The tracker is placed at the ankle location as it is considered favorable for recognising post-hip fracture rehabilitation activity movements [2] as represented in Fig. 3.

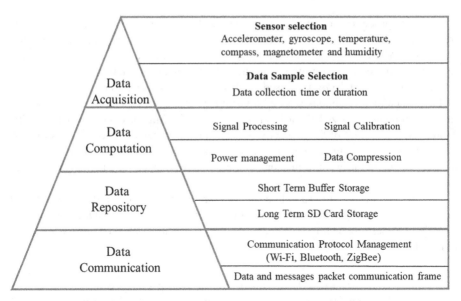

Fig. 2. Wearable monitoring tracker level key functionalities.

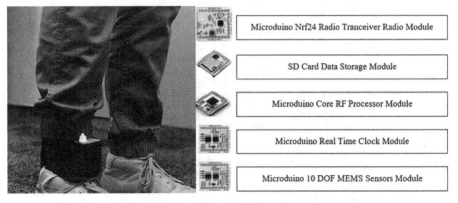

Fig. 3. Wearable tracker attached at ankle location and its module stack.

Among all the sensors available within the proposed tracker, only tri-axial accelerometer sensor is used. The use case implemented here is based on an algorithm that analyses the accelerometer data for recognising the hip fracture rehabilitation activity movement. Four different range of acceleration i.e. $\pm 2g$, $\pm 4g$, $\pm 8g$, $\pm 16g$ are offered by the sensor where g is the acceleration due to gravity in m/s^2. Acceleration range of $\pm 2g$ is selected as it is considered suitable for appreciating ambulatory activities relevant to the particular use case. The data is collected at a sampling frequency of 128 Hz [2].

As part of the preliminary experimental purpose, a young healthy participant was selected and provided with a wearable tracker. The participant was instructed to perform different sets of post-operative hip fracture rehabilitation activities as illustrated by in an ad-hoc manner for a time period of thirty minutes.

Raw and processed activity data storage space have been provided within a wearable tracker. For short term storage of the continually processed data, circular buffer has been used. Whereas SD card has a long-term storage purpose here. It can be used for long-term storage of the continuous raw activity movement accelerometer data.

An SD card of 64 GB was used in this research that can store data for around 30 days when run continuously for 24 hours a day. However, depending on the application requirement, any size SD card can be used for extending the data storage longevity. Moreover, availability of the raw activity data can aid clinicians or researchers for carrying further processing and confirmation to lower level analysis. The stored data can act as a backup in the event of misconnection or loss of connectivity to the gateway and the cloud.

Figure 4 represents the sample accelerometer activity data stored in the SD card respectively. The data packet format of the unfiltered data stored in the SD card comprises of node id, timestamp and triaxial (x, y and z axis) accelerometer readings as depicted in Fig. 4.

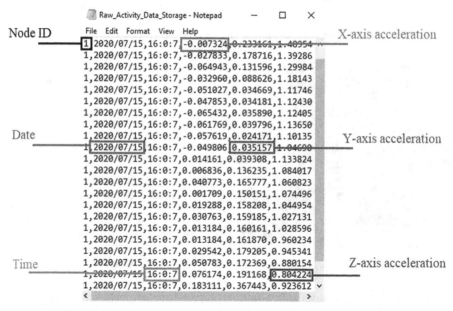

Fig. 4. Sample raw activity movement SD stored accelerometer data.

Figure 5 represents the 30-min trend of the raw activity movement data. From the small and large ripples observed across all the three axes, findings show that human subject is dynamic and is performing some type of activity movements. Moreover, there are situations where all the axes data is steady and linear which means subject is static and not performing any activity movements.

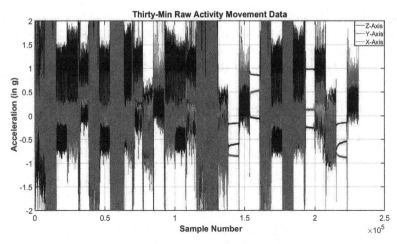

Fig. 5. Sample trend of the 30-min raw activity movement data.

After capturing the raw activity data, it is then subjected to filtering method. This is carried out by combing all the three axis samples that would eliminate tracker orientation problem, taking the mean, removing the DC offset and taking the average of every four samples. This would down-size the sampling rate to 32 Hz to comply with the 20 Hz suggested for everyday activities.

Communication can be established between the wearable device and the gateway node using different communication protocols like Wi-Fi, Bluetooth, or ZigBee. However, in this research Nordic nrf24 radio module has been used for data packet transmission and reception that works on an enhanced shock-burst protocol. The module supports three air data rates i.e. 250 kbps, 1 Mbps and 2 Mbps and is appropriate for ultra-low power wireless applications. Also, maximum of 32 bits size of data packet can be transmitted at a given data packet.

Point-to-point communication is established for transmission of activity movement data packet. The radio data packet is transmitted at a data rate of 250 kbps. For transmission and reception, radio pipe address is of 5-byte, 2 byte each for node id, packet trace, date, time and 4 bytes for processed data. The packet is transmitted once every second from the wearable tracker to the IoT gateway. One reading has a data packet size of 12 byte and 128 such packets are sent to the gateway containing 1536 bytes of data. The reason for sending it every four seconds is mainly related to the FFT process as the minimal time for activity detection without any loss of information or signal distortion. A portable Raspberry Pi (Rpi) attached with a nrf24 radio module is functioning as a gateway here (refer to Sect. 4.2).

Considering the constrained resources (data collection, processing and radio data packet transmission) available within a wearable tracker, it is important to investigate the energy consumption of the wearable tracker to observe how long the wearable tracker could be worn by a user when run continuously. The analysis has been done by comparing the energy consumption when tracker is in idle mode with that of fully functional operational mode.

Since Microduino module run on 3.3 V, the tracker is powered by a ½ AA recharge-able battery of 800 mAh at 3.7 V where the cut-off voltage is 2.75 V. The selection of the battery is random so that the tracker can operate for a full day. Table 1 represents the current in idle and operational (op) mode for each module used in the tracker [16].

Table 1. Wearable tracker modules current and power consumption [16].

S. No	Sensing modules	Idle mode current (mA)	Operational mode current (mA)
1	10 DOF	0.01	0.02–0.06
2	Nrf24	2.8	3–4.5
3	Core RF	22	22–24
4	SD card	1.5	5–7
5	RTC	0.032	0.05–0.1
Total current consumption		26.3 mA	30–36 mA
Total power consumption		97.4 mW	111–132 mW

From the practical measurement values provided by Table 1 above, a total current of 26.3 and between 30–36 mA is used by the tracker in idle and operating mode respectively. The total power consumed by both the modes are 97.3 and between 111–132 mW [16].

During transmission and reception, findings showed a minor fluctuation in the current consumption and is mostly 30–36 mA. This could be due to numerous reasons, but one potential reason is, it draws more current when the data is stored in the SD card. From the calculations, it is found that battery capacity is adequate to collect, store and transmit the data continuously for total duration of 22 h and must be recharged using a USB cable when a human subject is going to bed.

$$\text{Battery life of a wearable device} = 800\,\text{mAh}/36\,\text{mA} = 22.22 \approx 22\,\text{h} \qquad (1)$$

4.2 IoT Gateway or Edge Level Functionality

For IoT gateway or edge level functionality, a portable Raspberry Pi (Rpi) is connected through the serial communication port with a Microduino nrf24 radio module using serial peripheral interface (SPI) and is powered by two AA battery of 2500 mAh (i.e. equivalent to 5000 mAh) as shown in Fig. 6. The main purpose of making the device portable is to allow subjects to carry it anywhere and with ease while moving out of the allocated residence. However, other devices like smartphones, laptop and super gateway node can be used depending on the application requirements [16].

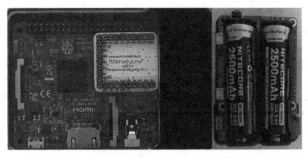

Fig. 6. Portable Raspberry Pi with Microduino nrf24 radio module top and bottom view.

This level provides the involvement of four key functionalities that could serve the purpose of overall rehabilitation activity movement monitoring post-operation as shown in Fig. 7.

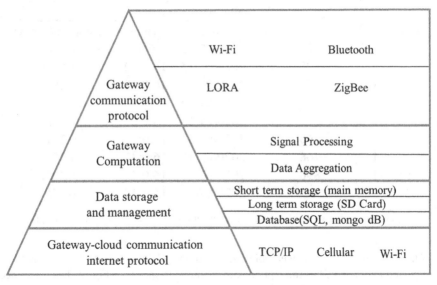

Fig. 7. IoT gateway or edge level key possible functionalities.

First is the wearable device gateway communication protocol that relates to the protocol used and as a protocol converter. This function helps in receiving the incoming data from the wearable device wirelessly and passing it through the serial communication. Second is the incoming data locally computed data storage and management. This can be short term storage available within the main memory (1 GB RAM), long-term storage in SD card (16 GB) and the data can be managed using database like MongoDB and MySQL. Third is the local computational capability analysed at the gateway level like signal processing and data aggregation. Before connecting to the cloud and using the fourth functionality i.e. cloud communication internet protocol like TCP-IP, cellular and Wi-Fi [16].

A complete 128 pieces of filtered data, representing the four second of data acquired by the wearable sensor is received regularly by the Rpi through serial communication. This incoming data packet is stored continually in the SD card residing within Rpi in form of text and csv file format. The screenshot of the data packet received at Rpi in csv formats is shown in Fig. 8. The data packet format comprises of Node id, packet trace count that increments by one and is used to keep a track which packet has been received or lost during the transmission, date, activity event and computed data value at wearable tracker level.

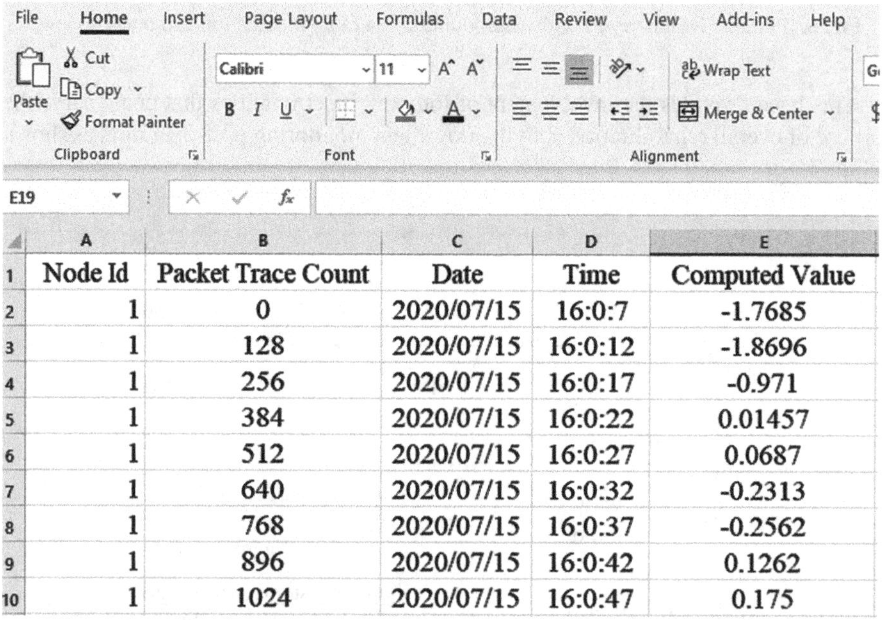

Node Id	Packet Trace Count	Date	Time	Computed Value
1	0	2020/07/15	16:0:7	-1.7685
1	128	2020/07/15	16:0:12	-1.8696
1	256	2020/07/15	16:0:17	-0.971
1	384	2020/07/15	16:0:22	0.01457
1	512	2020/07/15	16:0:27	0.0687
1	640	2020/07/15	16:0:32	-0.2313
1	768	2020/07/15	16:0:37	-0.2562
1	896	2020/07/15	16:0:42	0.1262
1	1024	2020/07/15	16:0:47	0.175

Fig. 8. Incoming wearable tracker data packet format received and stored in Rpi.

The representation of the wearable tracker computed data vs the five-minute activity time period event stored in the Rpi backup memory is shown in Fig. 9. The computed data graph is smoother and consistent compared to the raw activity movement graph as shown in Fig. 5. The smoothness and consistency are because of the pre-cleaned processing happening at the wearable sensor level. Across the graph, different ripples have been observed marked with different coloured circles that indicates subject has not been static all the time and has performed different types of activity movements. Moreover, a linear line marked with blue coloured circle indicates that subject was static. Therefore, it would be hard to discern which activity movement subject has performed based on the wearable tracker computed data. Hence, it requires further data computation and compression. This could be accomplished by using Fast Fourier Transform (FFT) based signal processing as discussed by [2]. The mathematical equations involved in this computational process are:

$$Maximum\,Amplitude\;(MA) = max|\beta_{128}(1:(5/Frequency\,Scale))| \qquad (2)$$

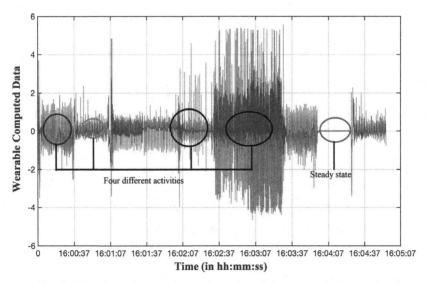

Fig. 9. Wearable computed data vs five-min activity time period event plot.

$$Frequency\ content\ (fMA) = (k-1) \times Frequency\ Scale \qquad (3)$$

β_{128} represents the 128 samples of the wearable computed data. $k = (1:5/Frequency\ Scale))$ where Frequency Scale = (data sampling frequency/D_4)/128. Here D_4 represents a value of four. It takes every fourth sample after removal of the DC offset of the collected accelerometer data. By taking every fourth sample, data sampling frequency is down sampled to 32 Hz to comply with the 20 Hz suggested for everyday activities [2].

Using the above equations, the process identifies maximum acceleration amplitude (MA) and frequency content of the maximum acceleration amplitude (f_{MA}) for each of the four seconds batch of data transmitted by tracker and received by Rpi. The timestamp of the final compressed data is associated with the end time of the activity movement sampling snap.

Based on the FFT computed data, activity threshold condition is set for a particular user based on the if-else condition. Hence, activity recognition is implemented at the gateway level based on MA and f_{MA} parameters. After recognising an activity, MA, f_{MA} and Recognised Activity Code (RAC) features are sent to the cloud [16]. Here, RAC denotes a number that ranges from 0–8 and is identified in Table 2. For example, is an activity recognised as swinging leg to a side, RAC of 5 will be sent to the cloud.

Along with the incoming wearable tracker data, final compressed data (MA, f_{MA} and RAC) is also stored in the Rpi SD card in form of a text and csv file. The sample of the final compressed data stored in Rpi is represented in Fig. 10.

Table 2. RAC for hip fracture rehabilitation activities [16].

S. no	RAC	Activity type
1	0	Static state
2	1	Slow walking
3	2	Fast walking
4	3	Leg movement
5	4	Lifting thigh upwards
6	5	Swinging leg to a side
7	6	Lying on back
8	7	Lying on stomach
9	8	Unrecognised activity

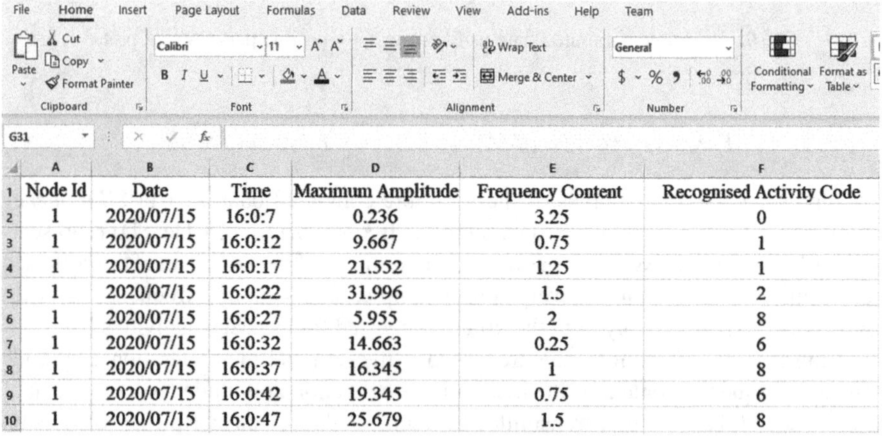

	A	B	C	D	E	F
1	Node Id	Date	Time	Maximum Amplitude	Frequency Content	Recognised Activity Code
2	1	2020/07/15	16:0:7	0.236	3.25	0
3	1	2020/07/15	16:0:12	9.667	0.75	1
4	1	2020/07/15	16:0:17	21.552	1.25	1
5	1	2020/07/15	16:0:22	31.996	1.5	2
6	1	2020/07/15	16:0:27	5.955	2	8
7	1	2020/07/15	16:0:32	14.663	0.25	6
8	1	2020/07/15	16:0:37	16.345	1	8
9	1	2020/07/15	16:0:42	19.345	0.75	6
10	1	2020/07/15	16:0:47	25.679	1.5	8

Fig. 10. FFT based signal processing data packet in csv format stored in Rpi SD card.

The stored data in the Rpi could be used to validate the packet loss and in case the connectivity to the cloud is lost, the activity movement data can still be recovered. The reason for storing the data within Rpi is because of the following reasons: First, to validate the data samples packet loss. Second, if the subject goes out of the allocated residence/rehabilitation care center or due to any other reason and the connectivity to the cloud is lost resulted. In this scenario, the incoming wearable tracker data and the activity recognition data can be recovered and sent to cloud once it finds the connectivity.

Thing Speak provides the capability for uploading the data in bulk where the limit of a single bulk update is up to 14400 pieces of data and the time limit between each sequential bulk update should be 15 s or more [17]. With the availability of this functionality, an algorithm flow chart is designed that represents the data transmission operation based on the internet connectivity establishment. This is shown in Fig. 11.

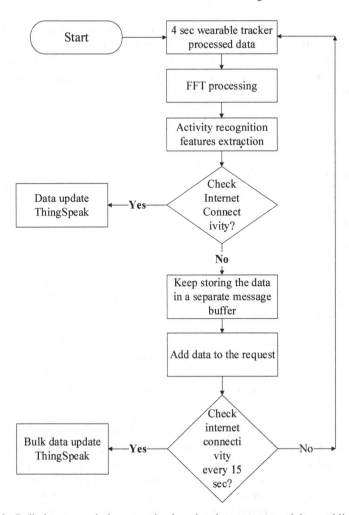

Fig. 11. Bulk data transmission operation based on internet connectivity establishment.

The algorithm starts by receiving the 4 s wearable tracker activity movement data. The data is then subject to FFT processing that extracts the activity recognition features (MA and f_{MA}). Following that the portable device checks for the internet connectivity. If connectivity exists, it updates ThingSpeak with the current data. However, if there is no connectivity, it keeps storing the data in a separate message buffer and add the data to request. After putting the data to request, it keeps on checking internet connectivity existence every 15 s. However, this time could be adjusted based on the application requirement. When it finds the connectivity, the complete data put to request is sent in bulk to ThingSpeak for an update. This process is executed repeatedly in loop. In this way, it will backtrack and fill the lost time activity movement data. To validate the algorithm and its functionality, simple experiment was conducted around a similar situation where subject was instructed to perform the rehabilitation activity movement in an outside environment for around 5 min where there is no internet connectivity and then come back to the lab to get connected to the internet to observe the bulk data upload to ThingSpeak. A sample illustration of such scenario is depicted in Fig. 12. It clearly represents that the 5 min data i.e. around 75 activity movement data points are uploaded in bulk to ThingSpeak.

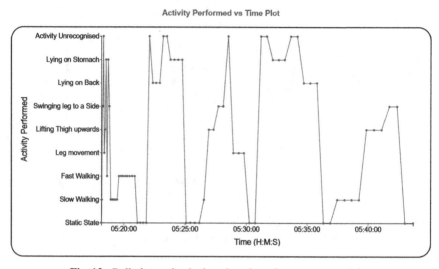

Fig. 12. Bulk data upload when there is no internet connectivity.

Another important aspect to consider along with the data packet reception, computation and sending of the data to the cloud, is to investigate the power consumption of the portable device. As mentioned earlier, portable gateway is powered by two AA battery of 2500 mAh. At 3.6 V. Rpi recommended input voltage is 5 V with a tolerance level of ± 5%. This means voltage between 4.75–5.25 could be supplied. Rpi3 current and power consumption when it is in idle and fully operational mode is represented in Table 3 [16].

Table 3. Rpi current and power consumption in idle and operational modes [16].

Rpi	Current consumption (mA)	Power consumption (W)
Idle mode	260	1.3
SD card file storage	285	1.425
Operational mode	670	3.35

Considering the operational mode current consumption of Rpi, calculations indicates that battery capacity is adequate to collect, store and transmit data continuously for around 7 h. Battery power is only needed when the subject is outdoor. As a result, 7 h should be enough to cover the data collection time before recharging again [16].

$$\text{Battery life of a Raspberry Pi3} = 5000\,\text{mAh}/670\,\text{mA} = 7.46 \approx 7\,\text{h} \qquad (4)$$

4.3 Internet-Cloud Level Functionality

Internet-Cloud level comprises five key functionalities and is represented by Fig. 13. Communication protocols like HTTP and MQTT can be used for data acquisition frame from the gateway or edge device. Cloud has its own data repository that can be used for storing the patient activity movement data or any other related knowledge data and can be managed at ease. With the use of the data available in the cloud repository, data computation techniques like digital signal processing, artificial intelligence and machine learning techniques can take place at different levels. In addition, cloud resources play significant role in data presentation, activity event detection, triggering a reaction in case of an emergency. Example commercially available tools are ThingSpeak and IBM analytics. The triggering of a reaction could be accomplished using different services like sending a text message or email and buzzing an emergency alarm so that immediate action can be taken [16].

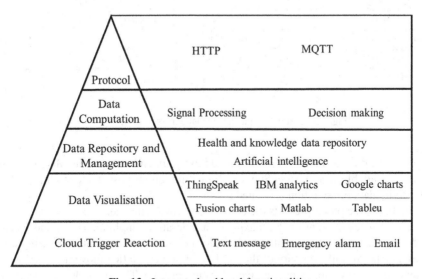

Fig. 13. Internet-cloud level functionalities.

For this research, ThingSpeak cloud platform has been used that collects and stores the data in real time. It allows developing IoT based processing and visualisation for the application. Computational tool like Matlab is integrated within the platform that could be used for any data computation and learning process. The usage of such tool could be significant in making more and precise sense out of the data as the computational resources are relevant to most of the operational requirements of the process.

The fundamental part of ThingSpeak relies in its communication channels where each channel accommodates a maximum of 8 fields of different data types, three location fields and one channel field for status value. It updates the data every one second and accommodate around 90,000 messages/day which also overcomes the lag associated in transmission of the processed data from the gateway to the cloud. However, other software's like Ubidots, IBM Watson and ThingWorx 8 can be integrated and facilitated within the system design based on the application requirements [16].

The final compressed data from the raspberry pi gateway (used within our implementation) is sent to the ThingSpeak using HTTP protocol. The data is spread across six different fields (Field 1: Node Id, Field 2: Date, Field 3: Time, Field 4: MA, Field 5: f_{MA}, Field 6: RAC) and is stored in the ThingSpeak cloud repository in three different formats i.e. JSON, XML and CSV format.

The sample screenshot of the data format stored in CSV format across field 4,5 and 6 can be seen from Fig. 14. In the figure, "created at" represents the date and time when the data is received by cloud. Entry id is created automatically by cloud as part of record for each field data transaction. Field 4, 5 and 6 represents the MA, f_{MA} and RAC respectively.

Field 4: MA			Field 5: f_{MA}			Field 6: ARC		
created_at	entry_id	field4	created_at	entry_id	field5	created_at	entry_id	field6
2020-07-15 07:03:32 UTC	1	0.236	2020-06-29 07:03:32 UTC	1	3.25	2020-07-15 07:03:32 UTC	1	0
2020-07-15 07:04:08 UTC	2	9.667	2020-06-29 07:04:08 UTC	2	0.75	2020-07-15 07:04:08 UTC	2	1
2020-07-15 07:04:54 UTC	3	21.552	2020-06-29 07:04:54 UTC	3	1.25	2020-07-15 07:04:54 UTC	3	5
2020-07-15 07:05:42 UTC	4	31.996	2020-06-29 07:05:42 UTC	4	1.5	2020-07-15 07:05:42 UTC	4	5
2020-07-15 08:28:11 UTC	5	5.955	2020-06-29 08:28:11 UTC	5	2	2020-07-15 08:28:11 UTC	5	8
2020-07-15 08:35:57 UTC	6	14.663	2020-06-29 08:35:57 UTC	6	0.25	2020-07-15 08:35:57 UTC	6	3
2020-07-15 08:38:07 UTC	7	16.345	2020-06-29 08:38:07 UTC	7	1	2020-07-15 08:38:07 UTC	7	4
2020-07-15 08:50:17 UTC	8	19.345	2020-06-29 08:50:17 UTC	8	0.75	2020-07-15 08:50:17 UTC	8	7
2020-07-15 08:59:38 UTC	9	25.679	2020-06-29 08:59:38 UTC	9	1.5	2020-07-15 08:59:38 UTC	9	2

Cloud created date and time   Cloud entry id

Fig. 14. Cloud data packet format across field 4, 5 and 6.

Using the data available within the cloud repository and utilizing the Matlab analytical tools available within ThingSpeak for computation purpose, the overall processed and activity data presentation is created represented in Fig. 15.

The first three plot represents the compressed parameters i.e. Maximum Amplitude (MA), Frequency content of the maximum acceleration amplitude (f_{MA}) and Recognised Activity Code (RAC) while the last plot i.e. human movement monitoring track represents the overall summary of the hip fracture rehabilitation movement performed by a young healthy subject over a given duration of time. The young healthy subject's activities that have been recognised are static, slow and fast walking, leg movement, lifting thigh upwards, swinging leg to a side and lying on stomach. The activity that was unrecognized is lying on back. This information offers near-real-time and trend monitoring to assist motivating the patient, help healthcare professionals in follow-up, emergency or decision making etc.

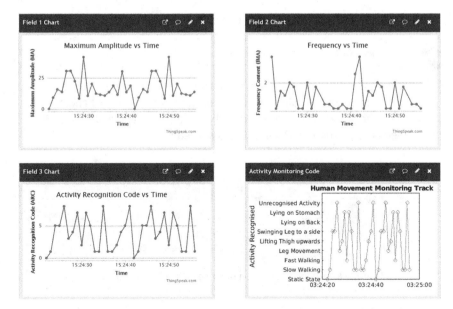

Fig. 15. Human movement monitoring cloud data presentation.

Moreover, with the available information, it is also essential to send alert text messages or email to the patient, their caretakers and the healthcare professionals in case of an emergency or essential follow-up. This would not only alert the required personal for an urgent follow-up or immediate action, but availability of such functionality is significant for the patient well-being, motivation and in gaining confidence. Hence, making them feel that the staff is there in case of a need and urgent situations.

ThingSpeak have plugins that provides the functionality of triggering a notification using ThingHTTP from IFTTT. IFTTT refers to "if this then that" and is a web service that allows to create applets which acts in response to another action [17].

A sample illustration of an automatic email sent to the patient using IFTT when no movement is observed for around 12 h. is represented in the Fig. 16. However, based on the application requirement different sets of conditions could be set and the system would respond to the query automatically either by sending an email or text message or both.

Therefore, the environment functionality was implemented successfully from all perspectives and in recognising most of the performed activities in real-time. However, further research work is required to test the system on maximum number of users to validate the user performance, its acceptability and usability of the proposed device. Another important aspect is to investigate how the system could be made personalized and adaptive to individual subject using deep learning techniques. A further investigate of the environment overall network and system performance is required especially when maximum number of users are connected and reporting to the same coordinator. An example of such scenario could be rehabilitation home or hospital.

The patient named X requires immediate follow up .   Inbox ×

Webhooks via IFTTT <action@ifttt.com> Unsubscribe
to me ▾

Dear Team, Patient X has been static for almost 12 hrs and requires immediate attention. Can you please follow up with the patient and the text message has also been delivered to both the patient and and their family members. Thank You, Patient Monitoring Team

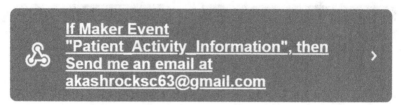

Fig. 16. Sample illustration of an email sent using IFTTT.

5 Conclusions

This paper proposed an IoT environment for monitoring human movements relevant to post-operative hip fractured patient rehabilitation process. Functionalities of the developed concept are tested based on activity data collected from a healthy young individual mimicking the targeted features. Considering the significance and role of each functionality, the proposed design can be made more generic to cater for wide range of human movement monitoring that could benefit healthcare applications. Experimental results showed the system capability in recognising the activity movements efficaciously. Further future work will investigate extending the concept for offering communal monitoring relevant for example to elderly care home. It will also investigate the role of artificial intelligence in big data analysis relevant to movement recognition and possibly movement pattern personalization.

References

1. W. H. O. (WHO). "10 Facts on ageing and health." https://www.who.int/features/factfiles/ageing/en/. Accessed May 2017
2. Gupta, A., Al-Anbuky, A., McNair, P.: Activity classification feasibility using wearables: considerations for hip fracture. J. Sensor Actuator Netw. **7**(4), 54 (2018)
3. W. H. O. (WHO). "Rehabiitation." https://www.who.int/news-room/fact-sheets/detail/rehabilitation. Accessed July 2019
4. Stucki, G., Bickenbach, J., Gutenbrunner, C., Melvin, J.: Rehabilitation: the health strategy of the 21st century. J. Rehabil. Med. **50**(4), 309–316 (2018)
5. Lee, I., Lee, K.: The Internet of Things (IoT): applications, investments, and challenges for enterprises. Bus. Horiz. **58**(4), 431–440 (2015)
6. Farahani, B., Firouzi, F., Chang, V., Badaroglu, M., Constant, N., Mankodiya, K.: Towards fog-driven IoT eHealth: promises and challenges of IoT in medicine and healthcare. Future Gener. Comput. Syst. **78**, 659–676 (2018)

7. Baek, J., Lee, G., Park, W., Yun, B.-J.: Accelerometer signal processing for user activity detection. In: Negoita, M.G., Howlett, R.J., Jain, L.C. (eds.) KES 2004. LNCS (LNAI), vol. 3215, pp. 610–617. Springer, Heidelberg (2004). https://doi.org/10.1007/978-3-540-30134-9_82

8. Sharma, A., Purwar, A., Lee, Y.-D., Lee, Y.-S., Chung, W.-Y.: Frequency based classification of activities using accelerometer data. In: 2008 IEEE International Conference on Multisensor Fusion and Integration for Intelligent Systems, pp. 150–153. IEEE (2008)

9. Karantonis, D.M., Narayanan, M.R., Mathie, M., Lovell, N.H., Celler, B.G.: Implementation of a real-time human movement classifier using a triaxial accelerometer for ambulatory monitoring. IEEE Trans. Inf. Technol. Biomed. 10(1), 156–167 (2006)

10. Sütő, J., Oniga, S., Buchman, A.: Real time human activity monitoring. In: Annales Mathematicae et Informaticae, pp. 187–196 (2015)

11. Nam, Y., Park, J.W.: Physical activity recognition using a single triaxial accelerometer and a barometric sensor for baby and child care in a home environment. J. Ambient Intell. Smart Environ. 5(4), 381–402 (2013)

12. Moschetti, A., Fiorini, L., Esposito, D., Dario, P., Cavallo, F.: Recognition of daily gestures with wearable inertial rings and bracelets. Sensors 16(8), 1341 (2016)

13. Kumari, P., López-Benítez, M., Lee, G.M., Kim, T.-S., Minhas, A.S.: Wearable Internet of Things-from human activity tracking to clinical integration. In: 2017 39th Annual International Conference of the IEEE Engineering in Medicine and Biology Society (EMBC), pp. 2361–2364. IEEE (2017)

14. Aminian, M., Naji, H.R.: A hospital healthcare monitoring system using wireless sensor networks. J. Health Med. Inform. 4(02), 121 (2013)

15. Mocnej, J., Seah, W.K., Pekar, A., Zolotova, I.: Decentralised IoT architecture for efficient resources utilisation. IFAC-PapersOnLine 51(6), 168–173 (2018)

16. Gupta, A., Al-Naime, K., Al-Anbuky, A.: IoT based testbed for human movement activity monitoring and presentation. In: ICT4AWE, pp. 61–68 (2020)

17. ThingSpeak. "ThingSpeak." https://thingspeak.com/. Accessed April 2020

Older Adults' Use of Whatsapp in a Polymedia Environment: Managing Timing, Content, Form and Practicality

Rhea Braunwalder[(⊠)], Julia Reiner, Cora Pauli, Veronika Hämmerle, and Sabina Misoch

OST Eastern Switzerland University of Applied Sciences, Rosenbergstrasse 59, 9001 St. Gallen, Switzerland
{rhea.braunwalder,julia.reiner,cora.pauli,veronika.haemmerle, sabina.misoch}@ost.ch

Abstract. We examine the media use in social relationship management of a group of highly educated and socially connected older adults aged 65+ in Switzerland. Based on a framework taking into account life-span theories of ageing and environmental factors we see older adults as active agents, shaping their social relationships in a polymedia environment. Drawing on empirical data we find that considering timing, content, etiquette and comfort guided our informants' choices according to situation and communication partner. It becomes clear that older adults consider their temporal and emotional resources in their interaction with others, in line with established life-span theories of ageing. WhatsApp has an especially positive and empowering significance, allowing spontaneous and easy communication of joyful messages between communication partners. The article contributes to research that combines established life-span perspectives on ageing with current environmental theories and provides evidence, that the needs, motivations and goals of older adults, as suggested by the socio-emotional selectivity theory and strategies used to reach these goals, as stated by the selection, optimization and compensation framework, remain unchanged in technologically shaped environments.

Keyword: Older adults · Social relationships · Polymedia · Whatsapp

1 Introduction

1.1 A Subsection Sample

As life expectancies and the proportion of older adults in industrialized nations rise, the importance of the social networks of older adults has increasingly come to the foreground [1]. Various studies have shown that social relationships are relevant for the well-being and health of people of all age groups [2] and health organisations increasingly raise attention to the correlations between social relationships and mental health in old age [3, 4]. Being integrated into a social network has been found to prevent illness and have positive effects on the health and life quality of older adults [1] and the Mental Health Foundation's report on relationships in the 21st century calls relationships "the forgotten foundation of mental health and wellbeing" [4].

Regarding social relationships of older adults, the much-cited socio-emotional selectivity theory (SST) [5, 6] is a life-span approach highlighting age-related changes in the motivations and goals of individuals. As individuals grow older, their motivational goals shift from gaining new experiences and information to experiencing positive emotions [6]. Negative experiences and emotions are weighted less and avoided, while positive emotions are more easily remembered and paid attention to [6]. The SST implies that older adults invest in emotionally meaningful social relationships and are better at emotional regulation in conflicts, social interactions and difficult situations [6]. Due to the limited perceived time left to live, instead of the quantity of relationships, the quality of relationships is regarded as important, and less close social ties are said to be neglected or even cut [6]. Thus, the social network of older adults is smaller and actively pruned and maintained.

The strategy of selecting social ties according to their emotional value can be brought into combination with the selection, optimization and compensation (SOC) framework [7], where selection consists of one of the three strategies older adults use to age well and deal with developmental changes in their abilities and resources. The two other strategies described by the framework are optimization, strategies used to improve or perform more efficiently and compensation, strategies used to deal with losses and burdens [7]. Both SST and SOC and are life-span developmental frameworks that consider individuals as active agents shaping their social relationships. The change of size and composition of social relationships and networks emerge not as inevitable consequences of ageing in terms of loss, but as based on decisions, motivations and goals actively pursued by individuals. For social relationships, this means older adults actively select which social relationships they invest time and effort in, as well as look for ways to improve, maintain and enhance relationships and compensate loneliness or other perceived burdens in their social networks.

Lifespan perspectives on ageing show that motivations and goals in the maintenance of social relationships change during our lifetime. However, the question of how our increasingly digital environment affects how we manage social relationships with multiple communication media and the influence of the technological environment in life-span frameworks as such has not been examined [8]. Further, older adults are often depicted as victims and losers of digitalization and studies examining the media use of older adults are often deficit oriented, rather than strengths and asset-based [9].

This article aims to combine individual-level theories on aging with current environment-related theories. We examine the use of communication media by older adults in a polymedia environment. This is done based on empirical data gained from a qualitative study on the WhatsApp use of older adults in Switzerland conducted in 2019 [10]. First, we describe the polymedia environment [11] we situate our findings in. After giving an overview of our study, context, and methods, we show how older adults use various communication channels and especially WhatsApp to construct and maintain their social relationships. We see older adults as active agents and focus on strengths and opportunities emerging through communication media use of older adults. We find that life-span perspectives on ageing, such as the SST [6] and SOC framework [7] remain decisive for the actions of older adults in polymedia environments.

2 Polymedia Environment

Next to individual-level factors described in the SST and SOC framework, gerontological research states that environmental factors influence ageing well [12]. Wahl, Iwarsson, and Oswald [12] propose a framework that integrates environmental factors to better assess the effects of an individual's technical environment on the aging process. They suggest that subjective, experienced-based belonging and behavior-based agency are essential to the way people interact with their environment [12]. However, they limit agency to "curiosity-oriented agency" (p. 310), and state that this type of agency decreases in age. According to the SST, the wish to belong and relate to other people is an emotional goal for older adults. If we see agency as behaving to achieve one's goals, then it may be assumed that emotion-oriented agency is present in old age [6]. Moreover, the framework alludes to technological developments in environments but does not give any indications of how our current environment can be theoretically conceived of. We suggest our setting can be situated in a polymedia environment [11], a term coined by Miller in his ethnography of interpersonal communication in transnational families.

In an earlier article on social relationships and information communication technology (ICT) (before the proliferation of the smartphone), Licoppe and Smoreda spoke of a "communication technoscape" [13] which included telephone calls, e-mails, SMS and messaging-services at the time just gaining in popularity. They described an emerging "ICT-based communication rationality", where individuals judge and interpret the form and content of an interaction in a framework of different options available to complete the task ([13], p. 4). They suggested that communication media do not replace each other but offer more diverse options for individuals to manage their social relationships and that social relationships are increasingly embedded in technoscapes [13].

More than ten years later, Madianou and Miller [11] examine a communication environment in which voice-calls, text messages and video calls can be used interchangeably on different platforms such as smartphones, tablets and computers at the desk or on the go. They consider different communication media as a landscape, in which the choice of communication media has emotional, social and moral consequences [11]. Here individuals take an active role and are guided in their choices by emotional needs and desires [14]. This state of polymedia can only exist if constraints such as costs, technological skills and accessibility of the concerned communication media do not play a decisive role anymore [11].

In her study of transnational Filipino families, Madianou [14] examines the use of smartphones between family members living apart. She describes smartphones as polymedia integrated into a larger polymedia environment encompassing other devices such as computers, laptops, and telephones. The decision of which communication channel to use turns into a message in itself. Smartphones, integrating multiple communication channels portably in one place, allow users to switch between communication channels with very little effort making it easier to choose from a range of communication channels to manage relationships [14].

To sum up our approach, in our study we examine how older adults' subjective feeling of belonging and agency to achieve emotional goals, as described by the SST and SOC, manifest in a polymedia environment with a special focus on WhatsApp and smartphone use.

3 Study Context

In Switzerland, the use of the mobile internet (on smartphones or tablets) has increased from 25% to 90% since 2010 [15], and 90% of the population owns a smartphone. This being said, in his study on the internet use of older adults in Switzerland, Friemel [16] states that the first-level digital divide regarding access and availability is still an issue especially for individuals aged 85+ and that social factors including income and education (but not gender) influence media use. This highlights the fact that older adults should not be regarded as a homogenous group as they differ regarding cognitive and physical health, income, educational background and social network type. Amongst the age group of 55 to 69-year-olds, 87% use a smartphone and reported using their smartphones most frequently to send and receive messages in 2018 [15]. The most popular application on smartphones for all age groups is WhatsApp [15], which is why we focus on this communication channel in particular. However, the polymedia lens allows us to not consider WhatsApp as a separate entity, but instead as a part of an integrated whole consisting of a range of other possible communication media.

Our empirical data consist of semi-structured interviews and ego-centered network maps of 30 adults aged 65+ in the German-speaking part of Switzerland. Data were generated in a study entitled "Effects of using WhatsApp on the subjective quality of social relationships of people 65+".[1] The semi-structured interviews focused on the WhatsApp use of participants on their smartphones. We asked about contents shared and not shared through WhatsApp, persons communicated with, usage history of WhatsApp, questions on other communication channels used, WhatsApp's influence on other communication channels, and the subjective experience of WhatsApp on the interviewee's social relationships.[2] Before the interview, the researcher and informant drew up an ego-centered network map listing all contacts of the informant, regardless of WhatsApp usage, on paper with post-its. The network map consisted of three concentric circles based on Kahn and Antonucci [17], positioning relationships to other people or groups from close to distant (emotional proximity). The roles, geographic proximity and frequency of contact were noted for each contact. Interviews were fully transcribed, and the data were analysed using qualitative content analysis [18].

Our sample included 15 men and 15 women aged between 66 and 84 (average age: 72.5). 22 informants had children, and 19 had grandchildren. Nine interviewees lived in

---

[1] The study was funded by the Swiss National Science Foundation, in a call addressing digital transformations in society. The participants were recruited through organisations for older adults and the institute's network. Sociodemographic data were recorded prior to the interview to ensure a homogenous sample regarding age and gender [10].

[2] The interviews were anonymized and transcribed and are accessible at https://doi.org/10.5281/zenodo.3753978.

single-person households. On average, the older adults named 23 social contacts, including friends, family and hobby and former work-related contacts. Informants reported regular contact with family and friends living nearby, and involvement in activities such as voluntary work, sports, language learning and cultural activities. None of our informants required notable instrumental support or had problems performing activities of daily living. Our informants' social networks could be classified as diverse-supported, family-focused, or friend focused-unsupported networks, as typologized by Fiori, Smith and Antonucci [19].[3] In sum, it can be said that our sample consisted of individuals of high socioeconomic status for Swiss circumstances, implying easy access to digital communication media, low financial constraints and technological literacy due to a supportive environment (friends and relatives), said to be decisive in the introduction of new technologies for older adults [20]. True to this, many described being motivated to use a smartphone by their close environment: friends who already used technological communication means, or children who gave them smartphones for their birthdays or Christmas and supported them in the use and acquisition of communication media. Courses and magazines where named as learning resources in technological communication, however with mixed results.

4 Communication Landscape

Although we set out to examine the use of WhatsApp and its effects on the subjective experience of social relationships of older adults in Switzerland, we found that rather than regarding WhatsApp as a separate communication means, many of the interviewed older adults mixed accounts of WhatsApp exchanges, e-mail and other communication channels. The means of communication mentioned by our informants were face-to-face meetings, phone calls (landline or smartphone), e-mails sent via computer or smartphone, SMS, Skype, instant-messaging (IM) services (WhatsApp, but also Viber and others), social network sites such as Facebook and letters or greeting cards. The different communication means were mentally categorized according to functions, comfort and distinct qualities each media possesses as the conversation with an 80-year-old widower shows:

Interviewee: "E-mail is like a monolog. You send something and get an answer. On the telephone, things are much more spontaneous. Right? Except for the pictures, you could put e-mail into the same basket as WhatsApp. It's only a back and forth, but little spontaneity. And if you're on the phone, well you hear the voice of the other person, right? That's great, that's worth more than…".[4]

Thus, instead of focusing on one communication media, in the following, we examine the management of relationships of older adults in a polymedia environment, describing concepts and showing examples of what guided the older adults' choice of communication media, if not cost, accessibility and skills.

---

[3] The types were: diverse-supported, family focused, friend focused-supported, friend focused-unsupported, restricted-nonfriends, unsatisfied, restricted-nonfamily-unsupported. They are based on data from the Berlin Aging Study, where the authors identified six network types for older adults, taking into account structure, function and quality of social networks.

[4] Quotations have been translated from Swiss-German to English by the authors. The original transcripts in High-German are available at https://doi.org/10.5281/zenodo.3753978.

4.1 Timing: Asynchronous by Choice

One aspect that was often mentioned in the conversations was the fear of bothering or disturbing other people. More broadly, this means taking into account the timing and frequency of contact. After considering the situation and the addressee, our informants chose the communication media to minimise the disturbance incurred on the counterpart. Whereas phone calls were seen as intrusive and demanding on the other people's time, IM services such as WhatsApp had the distinct advantage of leaving the other person the freedom to answer at their leisure. Choosing IM as a channel allowed the interviewees to feel less intrusive, more considerate of other people's time schedules, and experience more freedom in the disposition of their own time.

Not disturbing or imposing on others seemed a salient concern especially for our female informants. Clara,[5] aged 70 years old, described how compared to before when the only option was to call, she nowadays is more careful. Today, she chooses to send a WhatsApp message, which she perceives as less intrusive. She states, she sometimes does not want to be disturbed or does not feel like chatting on the phone with friends and prefers the efficient use of WhatsApp to send short and targeted messages. Berta, a widowed woman almost 80 years old, described how she experienced WhatsApp as liberating, and is now more communicative than before. While formerly, she constantly had the feeling of being a burden on someone, WhatsApp enables her to be more outgoing in the knowledge the counterpart can decide freely when and whether to answer. Nadine, aged 70 without children, described WhatsApp as a means to send cheerful messages without imposing on her friends. To two friends, who went through phases of illness, she regularly sent encouraging messages and felt closer and more connected to them in this way. She didn't make a difference between WhatsApp or SMS, both accessible through her smartphone, and felt that she would not have used the fix-line telephone to call or to achieve the same effect.

Jeanine, aged 68, lives with her husband and has two children with grandchildren living in the vicinity. She perceives her daughter as being so caught up with work and child-rearing, that she doesn't want to call her directly. Still, she likes feeling involved and being in touch with her family and extends invitations or sends pictures via a WhatsApp family group, keeping the door open for her children to reply in their own time.

These examples show how choosing to use WhatsApp as an asynchronous communication channel[6] allowed for more freedom on both sides and, that in contrast to younger user groups, who experience pressure to answer messages immediately and frustration when not receiving immediate replies [21], WhatsApp was regarded as a communication channel, where immediate replies were not expected. In line with the SST, the older adults were able to regulate their emotions and responses to others in relationships and did not expect immediate replies from their counterparts or feel pressured to answer messages immediately. Instead, they judged the importance of the situation and addressee before replying. They also knew of whom they could expect quick answers, and of whom they could wait several days before an answer came. They enjoyed their freedom to answer

---

[5] All names of the interviewed persons have been altered by the authors.

[6] Depending on the way of use, WhatsApp can be seen as an asynchronous or synchronous communication channel.

at will and felt in charge of their smartphone use. Sending WhatsApp messages could also be seen as a compensation strategy [7], compensating for loneliness due to time constraints and different schedules of close family members.

Hans, 68, a former lawyer living in a modern house with his wife described it like this: "The advantage of WhatsApp or SMS is of course, that it's immediate. You can do it immediately. If you think of something, you can get it done right then. And on the other side, as the recipient, I don't need to answer immediately but can answer later. That's why I think it's a simplification of the process. An optimization."

Choosing IM rather than a phone call, allows him to reach his goal, while not bothering his counterpart and transmits a feeling of higher efficacy for him. Different time schedules and constraints of family and friends can be accommodated. Using specific digital communication media is an optimization strategy, as described in the SOC framework [7], to maintain and enhance the relationship with selected contacts older adults want to invest time and resources in.

4.2 Content: Interesting and Joyful

A further notion regarded as important by the interviewed older adults was not related to the timing of messages, e-mails and calls, but rather to the content. Interest and positivity seemed guiding principles in communication, very much in line with SST, which states that older adults focus on relevant and positive emotions and memories and distance themselves from negative or irrelevant content [6]. Especially in the use of WhatsApp, many of our informants spent time evaluating whether the messages they wanted to send would be interesting, relevant and bring joy to their counterparts. The content of each message was carefully considered according to the situation and social relationship. In exchanges with friends, common interests were the main reason to exchange pictures, text messages, or articles. In exchanges with close family members, emotional pictures and positive joint memories were a common content of exchanges. Older adults reported that these exchanges heightened the subjective sense of closeness and belonging they had to close family members and friends, supporting results of studies showing that the need for relatedness is decisive for the intensity of use of WhatsApp [22]. Taipale and Farinosi found that short messages with low information content strengthen family ties and that WhatsApp can be used to care for other family members. It allows for fun intergenerational conversation, allowing each generation to choose their appropriate function and means of expression [23].

Clara reported exchanging pictures of plants and flowers with her childhood friend. Both know each other's interests and Clara believes sending her friend these pictures would bring her joy and would interest her. With a male friend, she exchanges newspaper articles which she reads and thinks he might appreciate reading too. By this, she consolidates her relationships with her friends. She feels WhatsApp is especially practical for this. Through these exchanges, she feels the relationships have become deeper and that she would not use different communication media to achieve this.

Negative feelings or memories in the use of WhatsApp, which for young people consisted of feeling watched, or surveilling other people, the fear of missing out and conflicts within romantic relationships and relationships with friends [22], were rarely mentioned by our informants. They reported it was annoying to receive too many irrelevant or inappropriate messages, especially in group chats with contacts more distant to them.[7] Here some older adults reported carefully considering which answers were relevant to which person and sending private messages instead of reverting to the group chat and negatively commented on other people's habits to carelessly respond to all group members. In choosing to send only interesting and relevant messages, the older adults maximized the effects of their messages, and invested time in relevant and emotionally positive relationship maintenance work.

4.3 Etiquette: Appropriate for Each Situation

In a polymedia environment, the choice of one communication channel over the other implies social, emotional, and moral consequences [11]. The older adults had a mental image of which channel was appropriate for which type of connection and content. Each message had a different value or was ranked in a hierarchy of valuable to worthless. However, expectations and rules were not explicit or the same for everyone. This was obvious mainly in intergenerational exchanges, but also exchanges between people of the same age group. The fact that WhatsApp offers different modalities, such as text- and voice-messages, voice-calls, video-calls, pictures, videos and emoticons allows individuals to fashion their messages as best suits them and may facilitate intergenerational communication in families, where each can communicate as they wish [23].

In the domain of value, it is important to broaden the field of examination and consider not only digital means of communication but all communication options available to older adults. Our informants naturally put digital communication means in relation to face-to-face meetings and handwritten correspondence such as letters and cards, and here it was very clear, that a face-to-face meeting was considered as irreplaceable by technological means. Receiving a text message instead of a more traditional card or looking at one's smartphone in the presence of others was judged as inappropriate. At the same time, sending and receiving pictures of holidays, grandchildren and everyday impressions was much appreciated and often named as an added value of using a smartphone and WhatsApp.

Martha, 68 years old, was one of our more radical informants. A widow with three children, she lives alone in a modern apartment. For her, face-to-face contact is the most valuable contact, and not replaceable by any other communication means. She prefers to use e-mail, but as her surrounding tends to use WhatsApp she uses it too, but strictly for information exchange. For her, WhatsApp is a quick and brief communication channel and she has very clear rules for the use of WhatsApp. She expects reactions to each of her messages and considers all else impolite. People who do not live up to her communication expectations, especially distant contacts, are deleted from her smartphone contact book and other channels and she also declines to see them in person. She deletes all messages after sending and receiving them and considers WhatsApp a means to an end. For her, it is clear: "And you have to take care yourself whether the contact is of good quality. You can't just attribute it to the system and believe, that just because I'm writing a certain amount of WhatsApp (messages), the relationship is good."

---

[7] These correspond to the 2nd and 3rd circles of their network maps.

Martha related an exchange with her son sending her the school-schedule of her grandchild which she occasionally takes care of via WhatsApp. She would have preferred her son to send her the schedule via e-mail or print it out and send it by post, which would have required more time from his side and does not count the message as a social contact. She went on to state that social contact means more than merely exchanging information via WhatsApp.

In general, when asked about the influence of WhatsApp on the quality of their relationships, most informants stated that WhatsApp might make maintaining relationships easier, be supportive and offer another option to exchange information and other messages with their contacts, but did not change the intensity or quality of the social relationship as such. This goes in line with the findings of Madianou [14], that polymedia and the use of smartphones could enrich and enhance the existing relationships of her informants, but could not create new relationships nor contribute to bettering difficult relationships. Instead, a solid basis for a relationship had to be there, which could then be nurtured by technological means.

Another interviewee was 67-year-old Jeremy. At the time of the interview, his father had recently died after a palliative-care phase. He described how he created a WhatsApp group with his brothers to manage the care of their father. After his father died, he deleted the group with his brothers and received condolence cards and messages on WhatsApp and via e-mail. He chose to answer only in the "traditional" way, by mail, carefully selecting an appropriate card for each person. Digital messages were judged by him as inadequate. The effort invested in sending messages "click, click" seemed inappropriate for the seriousness of the situation. In this context, the time and effort invested in sending a handwritten card made a card more valuable than a quickly sent message. He also pointed out how he was once added to a group that had been made during the sickness of his contact. This he felt was "too close" and he didn't feel WhatsApp was the right way to show closeness or compassion and left the group.

Hans often used the word "Wert" (value) in our interview. SMS never had a high "Stellenwert" (value, significance) for him, or it's not worth it to send someone a WhatsApp message, if you talk to the person on the telephone regularly, the "Mehrwert" (additional value) of the smartphone, is that it makes taking pictures and sending them easier. Presumably, subconsciously, he measured his communication actions, according to the effect they would have on his relationships. However, Hans went on to state, that although sending and receiving pictures gave him more insight into his contact's everyday life, he didn't believe that sending irrelevant pictures would especially intensify his relationship to a specific person.

Martha's rigorous approach includes deleting loose contacts who do not reply to her messages in the time expected. She feels if they do not invest time and effort into the relationship it is not worth it to do the same for them. She doesn't want any contacts in her phonebook who are not looking for a personal relationship with her. She wants to "keep it clean" and doesn't care about the mere amount of contacts she has. This is in contrast with the way younger adults, according to the SST [6] seek to increase their horizons and acquire new friends.

As in the chapter above, the examples indicate that both senders and receivers had a notion of what time and effort invested in a relationship and an act was appropriate and that the expectations were not always the same on both sides.

4.4 Comfort: As Easy as Possible

Other factors important in considering which communication channel to use were comfort, practicality and ease of use. While sending e-mails was practical for long messages with attachments, documents that should be printed out and links, telephone calls were practical for matters where an immediate reply was needed from a specific person or for more emotional and complex exchanges. Especially e-mail used on a personal computer (booting up the device), or a telephone (constrained to one place) implied time and effort. WhatsApp and Smartphones were considered as especially easy and quick to use, which might describe why they are so readily adapted into their communication patterns. Often stated practical uses of WhatsApp were organising events such as birthday parties, dinners, and trips in group chats.

Frederick, a 70-year-old man living with his wife, uses a WhatsApp group to organise weekly billiard meetings with his two friends. He also has a WhatsApp group with his wife, sons and daughters in law to manage the use of their joint holiday home. He describes how practical WhatsApp is compared to the telephone to coordinate events or meetings with groups. The exchanges in the group are purely functional and kept short. When asked what he would do, if WhatsApp ceased to exist, he merely stated he would go back to using the telephone. For many of our informants, the advent of new communication channels led to a shift in the used communication media, but not to a shift in the quality of the social relationships as such.

WhatsApp as a tool is perceived as efficient, goal-oriented, supportive and useful. Especially being able to take pictures with the smartphone and send them to others using WhatsApp is a strong point. Further, WhatsApp is practical to keep in touch with more distant contacts such as holiday acquaintances, former friends, or other loose contacts. Sending a greeting to a close family member, a quick message to say "I'm thinking of you" is possible without further ado, and people who are on holiday or living abroad in a different time-zone can more easily be reached. However, our informants stated it could not replace the physical presence of another person.

Acquaintances who are not so close but have the potential to become close contacts can be communicated with, without investing too much time and effort, thus decreasing the loss if the relationship turns out to be irrelevant.

Rita, 72, living alone, described how she has been starting to communicate with the mother of her son's fiancée: "Well, I haven't known her since a long time. At that time WhatsApp already existed. But I still think, if we would have to talk on the phone, they are also retired and on the move a lot, the two of them, her husband and herself, and I am also up and about. So, if we would talk on the phone, we would have to schedule it to the early morning, or evening. And WhatsApp is direct. You can write the moment you experience something. Or when you have the time for it, and I feel that is practical."

Instead of having to plan and save time for communication, she can send messages on the go, whenever she has time. Maintaining this new relationship becomes easier, as it requires less effort and planning on both sides. The ready incorporation of new media, in this case, WhatsApp, into the polymedia environment of our informants, is an indicator of the optimization strategies [7] older adults put into place while managing social relationships.

5 Conclusion and Discussion

In this article, we examine the media use in social relationship management of a group of highly educated and socially connected older adults in Switzerland. Based on a framework taking into account the subjective feeling of belonging, purposeful behaviour and environmental factors [12], we see older adults as active agents, shaping their social relationships in a polymedia environment.

Our informants considered different communication media in an integrated environment consisting of voice-calls, video-calls, e-mails, IM (WhatsApp or others), SMS, letters and cards. This indicates that the environment can be considered a polymedia environment where communication media do not replace each other, but rather offer more options with which people can manage their social relationships. Access, availability and skills, although not irrelevant, are not the main determinants of the use of communication technologies. Instead, we found that considerations of timing, content, etiquette and comfort guided our informants' choices according to situation and communication partner (see also Table 1). Moreover, in line with life-span theories of ageing, it became clear that older adults carefully weighted their temporal and emotional resources in their interaction with others. In this polymedia environment, WhatsApp, with its different modalities, has an especially positive and empowering significance, allowing spontaneous and easy communication of joyful messages between different communication partners. The use of the smartphone might be seen as a tool to make managing social relationships easier and more comfortable, lowering the threshold to contact others and offering more possibilities to invest time in relationships otherwise neglected.

The article contributes to research that combines established life-span perspectives on ageing with current environmental theories and provides evidence that the needs, motivations and goals of older adults, as suggested by the SST and SOC framework, remain unchanged in technologically shaped environments.

As our sample included people with diverse-supported, family-focused and friend focused-supported network types, further research should include a more diverse sample as well as unsupported and restricted network types. It could be examined if the state of polymedia occurs in these cases and if the considerations made, when communicating with others, differ between network types. Examining less well-off and physically impaired older adults, could give insight into mediated compensation strategies [7] put into place by older adults and confirm our proposition, that the SOC and SST remain valid in polymedia environments.

Another fruitful research topic could be to examine the expectations and implicit communication rules or "rationales" [13] that exist when using communication technology, how these emerge and how they differ according to social network type and age. Further studies could go on to examine social consequences of the polymedia environment, such as changes in family care relationships at a broader level, consequences and potentials at a community level and also gender-related consequences of technology

Table 1. Simplified communication landscape, compiled by the authors.

	e-Mail	WhatsApp	SMS	Telephone	Letters/cards	Face-to-face meeting
Timing	Asynchronous	Asynchronous and synchronous, spontaneous	Asynchronous	Synchronous, arranged in advance or potentially disturbing	Planned in advance	Planned in advance
Content and quality	Information (News, Articles, Schedules)	Joyful and entertaining exchanges, pictures, videos, light content, organizational matters	Short informational messages	Longer talks, might be boring, deeper exchanges between friends, catching up, can hear other person's voice	Hand-written greetings, emotional content	Hearing and seeing the other person, seen as the most valuable type of social contact, basis of a relationship
Appropriate for	Longer and more complex texts, attachments, work related matters	Greetings, organizing events, fun and light exchanges, geographically distant people		Personal and private matters, urgent matters	Special occasions, deaths, birthdays, anniversaries	Personal, private, and sensitive matters, exchanges
Comfort	Bound to a desktop, time needed to boot the computer, keyboard more comfortable for long messages, screen larger for reading long texts	Portable and mobile, but small keyboard not practical for long messages,	Implies costs	Only at home, might be fixed to a place (cable)	Preparation needed: buying a card, writing it, bringing it to the post	Travel to meeting point might be required
Social relationships	Third circle (Work, Hobby)	Predominantly first circle (close family and friends), intergenerational	First and second circle	First circle (friends)	First circle (close family and friends)	First and second circle

use, which has often been examined in developing countries (for example [24]), but less so in industrialised nations. Further, showing older adults how communication media can help them reach emotional goals could empower and motivate them to close the "digital divide". By connecting digital communication with older adults' life experiences and social, cultural and personal resources, the development of community and family-based support systems could be enhanced. This would contribute to a society, where older adults feel included and supported in technology use.

References

1. Ellwardt, L., Hank, K.: Soziale Netzwerke im Alter. In: Hank, K., Schulz-Nieswandt, F., Wagner, M., Zank, S. (eds.) Alternsforschung. Handbuch für Wissenschaft und Praxis, 1st edn., pp. 339–356. Nomos, Baden-Baden (2019)
2. Antonucci, T.C., Ajrouch, K.J., Birditt, K.S.: The convoy model: explaining social relations from a multidisciplinary perspective. Gerontologist (2014). https://doi.org/10.1093/geront/gnt118

3. Bachmann, N.: Soziale Ressourcen. Förderung sozialer Ressourcen als wichtiger Beitrag für die psychische Gesundheit und eine hohe Lebensqualität, Bern (2020)
4. Relationships in the 21st Century. The forgotten foundation of mental health and well-being, London (2016). https://www.mentalhealth.org.uk/sites/default/files/Relationships-in-21st-century-forgotten-foundation-mental-health-wellbeing-full-may-2016.pdf. Accessed 13 Aug 2020
5. Carstensen, L.L., Isaacowitz, D.M., Charles, S.T.: Taking time seriously: a theory of socioemotional selectivity. Am. Psychol. **54**, 165–181 (1999)
6. Carstensen, L.L., Fung, H.H., Charles, S.T.: Socioemotional selectivity theory and the regulation of emotion in the second half of life. Motiv. Emot. (2003). https://doi.org/10.1023/A:1024569803230
7. Baltes, P.B., Brim, O.G. (eds.): Life-Span Development and Behavior, vol. 3. Academic Press, New York (1980)
8. Schulz, R., Wahl, H.-W., Matthews, J.T., de Vito Dabbs, A., Beach, S.R., Czaja, S.J.: Advancing the aging and technology agenda in gerontology. Gerontologist (2015). https://doi.org/10.1093/geront/gnu071
9. Doh, M.: Heterogenität der Mediennutzung im Alter. Theoretische Konzepte und empirische Befunde. Gesellschaft - Altern - Medien, vol. 2. kopaed, München (2011)
10. Hämmerle, V., Pauli, C., Braunwalder, R., Misoch, S.: WhatsApp's influence on social relationships of older adults. In: Proceedings of the 6th International Conference on Information and Communication Technologies for Ageing Well and e-Health – ICT4AWE, vol. 1, pp. 93–98 (2020). ISBN 978-989-758-420-6. https://doi.org/10.5220/0009470100930098
11. Madianou, M., Miller, D.: Polymedia: towards a new theory of digital media in interpersonal communication. Int. J. Cult. Stud. (2013). https://doi.org/10.1177/1367877912452486
12. Wahl, H.-W., Iwarsson, S., Oswald, F.: Aging well and the environment: toward an integrative model and research agenda for the future. Gerontologist (2012). https://doi.org/10.1093/geront/gnr154
13. Licoppe, C., Smoreda, Z.: Are social networks technologically embedded? Soc. Netw. (2005). https://doi.org/10.1016/j.socnet.2004.11.001
14. Madianou, M.: Smartphones as polymedia. J. Comput.-Mediat. Commun. (2014). https://doi.org/https://doi.org/10.1111/jcc4.12069
15. Media Use Index 2018, Zürich (2018). www.media-use-index.ch. Accessed 2 Oct 2019
16. Friemel, T.N.: The digital divide has grown old: determinants of a digital divide among seniors. New Media Soc. **18**, 313–331 (2016)
17. Kahn, R.L., Antonucci, T.C.: Convoys over the life course: attachment, roles, and social support. In: Baltes, P.B., Brim, O.G. (eds.) Life-Span Development and Behavior, vol. 3, pp. 253–286. Academic Press, New York (1980)
18. Mayring, P.: Qualitative Inhaltsanalyse. Grundlagen und Techniken, 12th edn. Beltz, Weinheim (2015)
19. Fiori, K.L., Smith, J., Antonucci, T.C.: Social network types among older adults: a multidimensional approach. J. Gerontol. Psychol. Sci. **62B**, 322–330 (2007)
20. Kamin, S.T., Lang, F.R., Kamber, T.: Social contexts of technology use in old age. In: Kwon, S. (ed.) Gerontechnology. Springer, New York (2016). Doi: https://doi.org/10.1891/9780826128898.0003
21. Church, K., de Oliveira, R. (eds.): What's up with WhatsApp? Comparing mobile instant messaging behaviors with traditional SMS. In: Proceedings of the 15th International Conference on Human-Computer Interaction with Mobile Devices and Services. ACM (2013)
22. Karapanos, E., Teixeira, P., Gouveia, R.: Need fulfillment and experiences on social media: a case on Facebook and WhatsApp. Comput. Hum. Behav. **55**, 888–897 (2016)

23. Taipale, S., Farinosi, M.: The big meaning of small messages: the use of WhatsApp in inter-generational family communication. In: Zhou, J., Salvendy, G. (eds.) ITAP 2018. LNCS, vol. 10926, pp. 532–546. Springer, Cham (2018). https://doi.org/10.1007/978-3-319-92034-4_40

24. Chew, H.E., Ilavarasan, V.P., Levy, M.R.: Mattering matters: agency, empowerment, and mobile phone use by female microentrepreneurs. Inf. Technol. Dev. (2015). https://doi.org/10.1080/02681102.2013.839437

Use of a Socially Assistive Robot to Promote Physical Activity of Older Adults at Home

Esther Ruf[(⊠)] ⓘ, Stephanie Lehmann ⓘ, and Sabina Misoch ⓘ

Institute for Ageing Research, OST Eastern Switzerland University of Applied Sciences,
Rosenbergstrasse 59, 9001 St. Gallen, Switzerland
esther.ruf@ost.ch

Abstract. Demographic change is leading to a higher proportion of older adults. The health and care sector must adapt because diseases and functional limitations increase with age. Strategies are required to promote and improve the functional capacity of older adults. A key factor in protecting health is regular physical activity. However, older adults do not move enough. It is therefore important to develop strategies to encourage older adults to be physically active. Regular motivation and guidance are helpful, but often not feasible due to staff shortages and high costs of personalized trainers. One solution is to use technology. Several studies have shown the positive effects of robots as instructors and motivators for physical activity. However, it has not been examined whether it is suitable in the private household. Therefore, the explorative user study investigated whether a socially assistive robot could be a practical solution to motivate older adults living independently to exercise regularly. Seven older adults participated. They trained one week with the robot as an instructor. The participants enjoyed the robot, but some technical difficulties such as slowness, communication, face recognition, stability, and acoustic problems occured. The participants experienced the robot as motivating, but they expected habituation effects. Even if the robot used was not suitable for autonomous training at home, this research can help find new ways to motivate older adults to engage in regular physical activity and improve technical solutions with the involvement of older adults.

Keyword: Robot · Physical activity · Older adults

1 Background

1.1 Societal Changes

Worldwide, the percentage of older adults is increasing [78]. In Europe, 19.4% of the population were aged over 65 in 2017. This percentage is expected to reach 28.5% in 2050 [21]. The percentage of older adults over 80 years will double to 13% from 2019 to 2070 [15]. In Switzerland, the percentage of people over 65 years is 18.9% in 2020 and is expected to rise to 25.6% until 2050 [24].

To deal with Europe's ageing society, health and care systems must adapt and provide a long-term vision for well-functioning and resilient public health systems, in particular

© Springer Nature Switzerland AG 2021
M. Ziefle et al. (Eds.): ICT4AWE 2020, CCIS 1387, pp. 78–95, 2021.
https://doi.org/10.1007/978-3-030-70807-8_5

by investing in disease prevention [16]. To be able to benefit from the prolonged life span, healthy aging is important, which includes good physical and mental health. Therefore, the ability to acquire and maintain skilled motor abilities to adapt to the challenges and requirements of the changes in daily life is highly relevant [30]. However, with increasing age, the incidence of diseases and functional limitations also increases. There is a substantial increase in physical problems that affect the performance of activities for daily living (ADLs) due to physical and medical problems associated with age [44], and the number of people with severe cognitive disabilities in 2050 will be three times larger than today [1, 87]. In Switzerland 5.7% of the 65 to 79-year-olds have problems in activities of daily living (ADL) and 15.9% of those over 80 [22]. 24.8% of the 65 to 79-year-olds have problems with instrumental activities of daily living (IADL) and 55.9% of those over 80 [23]. Aging societies must therefore develop effective strategies to promote and improve the functional capacity of older adults to maintain physical and cognitive health and therefore their participation in social life.

1.2   Physical Activity of Older Adults

It has been shown that physical activity is age-dependent: there is a decrease in physical activity with increasing age [5], and motivation for physical activity decreases with age [63], so many older adults do not move enough [38, 83]. Older adults living at home have a high incidence of falls, due to a sedentary lifestyle, deconditioning, and comorbidities [68]. The prevalence of pre-frail and frail syndrome is estimated high in older adults [8]. Further, older adults are found to be the population subgroup with the highest levels of sedentary time [91] and the lowest levels of physical activity [74]. This has various negative effects like reduction in (functional) everyday abilities [81], losses in health, self-confidence, and self-efficacy, reduced participation in social life, decrease of cognitive abilities, and increased loneliness [e.g. 5, 27, 31]. Therefore, there is a high need for healthcare systems to develop effective solutions to ensure the physical wellbeing of older adults [10]. Besides the positive effects of activity on physical health, Tully et al. [76] showed that replacing 30 min of sedentary behavior with light or moderate physical activity was associated with improved anxiety symptoms in older adults.

Physical exercises have a very positive impact on overall health status and cognitive health [90]. There is strong evidence that regular physical activity is associated with comprehensive benefits of older adults [2, 11] and also mental health [64, 65, 76].

As a central protective factor for health, regular physical activity shows the most stable evidence of benefits in terms of health and independence in old age [9]. It has positive effects on physical complaints [28], and can reduce the occurrence of falls [52, 70]. Frailty can be reduced by targeted physical training [e.g. 42], and quality of life and independence can be increased [e.g. 13].

The ability to walk safely in one's environment facilitates a physically and socially active life and access to goods and services [60]. Furthermore, regular physical activity can reduce the risk of high blood pressure, stroke, diabetes, cancer, or depression [88, 90]. Besides positive effects on physical health, movement exercises also have measurable positive effects on cognitive performance [51]. Physical exercise is one of the possible treatments for depressive mood which is especially important in old age as there is a high prevalence of depression in older adults [32, 53, 61]. Therefore, one of the most important fields of action is the promotion of physical activity in old age [83] with direct positive effects for the older population and at the societal level by preventing a further increase in health costs due to illness and care.

To ensure and support active aging, many countries have invested in promoting activities. Via media platforms, they provide physical exercises for older adults that they can perform at home. The exercises are specifically designed to attend to age-related limitations and to improve the health of older adults. For example, Pro Senectute Switzerland [56] has designed sets of physical exercises that older adults may perform at home to improve their strength, flexibility, and balance [71].

However, the difficulty is to get older adults to integrate physical exercises into their daily lives. Information campaigns highlight the benefits of physical activity for older adults and various exercise programs are specifically designed to promote physical activity among older adults. But the problem often is to motivate older adults to perform the exercises regularly. Exercise programs are beneficial only when done regularly and over a longer period [28]. Regular invitation and guidance seem to be helpful [39] and to be more effective than unguided training [29].

There are possibilities to ensure regular training, for example with a homecare assistant which is quite costly, or going to a group training what requires traveling, what could be a barrier for some older adults living in rural areas or having to travel with public transportation. These solutions do not apply to the growing number of older adults that need assistance but still living in their own home. Older adults express the wish to be able to age independently in their familiar living environment for as long as possible [33], which is in line with the concept of "ageing in place" [43]. Older adults are nowadays living longer in their own homes [17] but at the same time, the lack of nursing staff is increasing [46, 47, 89]. Therefore, an alternative must be found.

1.3 Use of Technology as One Possible Solution

There is a lack of resources and personnel to meet these societal challenges. So, solutions that promote the health of older adults and support them to live independently at home are of considerable interest. The question is whether the use of technology can contribute to enhance independence and therefore reduce individual and societal costs of caring by preventing disability and frailty of older adults [77]. The technological advances could provide additional solutions to meet these social and individual challenges [66]. Amongst these, socially assistive robots could be used in everyday living environments and for example advise older adults in performing exercises at home and increase the motivation of older adults to do so. In this way, the autonomy of older adults could be maintained, and their well-being could be increased, carers could be relieved physically and psychologically, and costs could be saved.

Based on their application, robots can be divided into industrial robots (robots for manufacturing) and service robots (robots for services). In the case of service robots as a separate subclass of robots, the focus is on the direct benefit to humans. The International Organization for Standardization defines a service robot as a robot "that performs useful tasks for humans or equipment excluding industrial automation applications (ISO 8373)" [36].

In the field of assistive robotics, different types of robots have been developed that perform various activities with the aim to maintain healthy life habits of older adults by engaging their users to develop training activities in physical and mental activities and rehabilitation, including humanoid robots, exoskeletons, rehabilitation robots, service robots, and companion-type robots [55]. According to the categorization of assistive robots for elderly of Broekens, Heerink, and Rosendal [7], assistive robots can be divided into rehabilitation robots (e.g. wheelchairs and exoskeletons) and socially assistive robots, with the subcategories service robots and companion robots (p. 94 ff). In their review of robots supporting elderly people with no cognitive decline, Bedaf, Gelderblom & DeWitte [3] identified 107 robots for the elderly in their home situation to prolong independent living. Nowadays, commercially available robots focus on the physical support of self-care related activities. Most of the robots in the development phase claim to physically support mobility-related activities. Few robots in the development phase focus on providing physical support for self-care related activities.

In some studies, a robot was used as an exercise coach for older adults. The motivation of older adults was positively influenced by socially assistive robots [75] to stay active via social exercise encouragement [19, 37] and it was more motivating to perform physical activity with a robot than alone [86] or with a standard training plan [85] and the effort was boosted with a humanoid robotic partner compared to exercising alone [62]. Shen and Wu [69] even found a preference for robotic instructors over human instructors.

Although several studies found positive effects of socially assistive robots as instructors and motivators for physical exercise for older adults, it is not yet tested if a robot as a fitness coach is suitable in private households, where physical exercises have to be performed independently with the robot.

Therefore, the question of this project was whether a socially assistive robot that acts as a training coach could be a practical solution to motivate older adults living independently at home to exercise regularly. It was analyzed in an explorative user study.

2 Methods

2.1 Participants

Older adults were recruited via the network of senior citizens of the institute. For inclusion, the participants had to be over 65 years, with no physical or cognitive restrictions, living in private homes in Switzerland, and German-speaking. Eight older adults could be enrolled in the study.

2.2 Exercise Program

In a program called "Walk safely, stand safely" Pro Senectute Switzerland [56] compiled exercises for daily exercises, consisting of three strength exercises, three standing balance exercises, and three walking balance exercises with each exercise having an easier and a harder version [71]. For the present study, three strength exercises and three balance exercises were selected out of the original nine exercises. The selection was made based on the capabilities of the socially assistive robot. The six exercises were presented in three versions: (1) a programmed humanoid robot (NAO V6, 6th version) that performed the exercises as an autonomous fitness coach; (2) written instructions and pictures of the exercises based on the official booklet of the campaign from Pro Senectute Switzerland; (3) a video tutorial based on the official video of the campaign. The version of the exercise program shown by the socially assistive robot, with an introduction and six exercises with verbal instructions lasted 36 min (for details see [6]).

2.3 Questionnaire

To examine whether a socially assistive robot is practical to be a training coach and motivate older adults to exercise, a questionnaire was compiled consisting of the items shown in Table 1.

Table 1. Overview of used variables.

Variable	Item	Source
Sociodemographic	Age in years Gender Marital status Type of housing Former professional activities Level of education Residential area	Self-developed with recommendations from Flandorfer [25]
Health status	General Health	Short Form Health Survey, SF-36 [82]
Current physical activity	Frequency in one week Duration of one session Social aspect (alone/group)	Self-developed
Self-efficacy	Rely on own skills Mastering problems by myself Solving complicated tasks	Allgemeine Selbstwirksamkeit Kurzskala (ASKU) [4]
Technical affinity	Interest in technology Interest in new technology	Adopted questions from Seifert and Meidert [67]
Socially assistive robot as an exercise coach in older adult's homes	Regularity Difficulties Fun Motivation Operation Own experience Recommendations	See Table 2 [based on 18–20, 75, 85, 86]

At the end of the study, all participants were asked seven questions in a qualitative semi-structured interview about the exercises with the socially assistive robot (see Table 2). We used qualitative methods to identify important issues and understand subjective opinions and problems in-depth [49].

Table 2. Questions in the qualitative semi-structured interview.

Questions
(1) Were you able to exercise regularly (3 times a week) with the robot NAO?
(2) Were there any difficulties during training? What did not work?
(3) Was it fun to train with the robot?
(4) Was it motivating for you to train with the robot NAO?
(5) How was the operation of the robot for you? Were there any difficulties?
(6) If you look at your own experiences, do you think the use of NAO for older adults to activate movement is possible in principle?
(7) Would you like to tell us anything else about your experience with the robot?

2.4 Procedure

The study ran for 12–14 weeks for each participant from June 2019 to December 2019. The participants first had an individual introduction at the study center where they signed the informed consent form. Questions (T0) about sociodemographic factors, physical training, state of health and self-efficacy were asked before the participant was introduced to all three conditions (robot, booklet, video). After this first training with the socially assistive robot to get used to the handling, commands, etc. (see Fig. 1) the participants were asked questions about the robot as a fitness coach (T1). The participant was instructed to place the robot on the floor and not on a table due to its instability to avoid a fall and thus damage to the robot. Figure 2 shows the survey dates and used instruments.

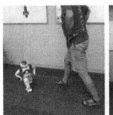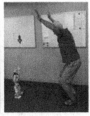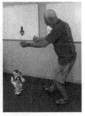

Fig. 1. First contact of an older adult with the robot in the study center. Image source [6] (published in [58]).

According to a predetermined schedule, each participant then carried out the training independently at home. The participant exercised one week with each version of instruction (with robot (Condition Robot; CR), with booklet (Condition Booklet; CB), with video (Condition Video; CV)). In the training week, the participant should perform the six movement exercises three times. After each training week, the participant had to fulfill a study protocol. Between the one-week training in each condition the participants had a two-week break (B) in which they were not allowed to perform the six exercises.

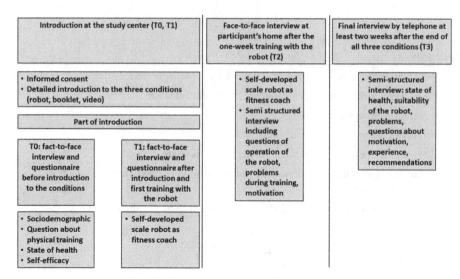

Fig. 2. Survey dates and used instruments.

Figure 3 summarizes the procedure of the study. A face-to-face interview was conducted immediately after the one-week training with the robot at the participants' private home (T2). The final interview was conducted by phone (T3) two weeks after the last training week (see Figs. 2 and 3). The sequence in which the participants went through the three conditions varied to avoid order effects. Due to a technical failure of the robot and the fact that the repair took longer than the planned break, it was not possible to realize the same break time between the conditions for all participants.

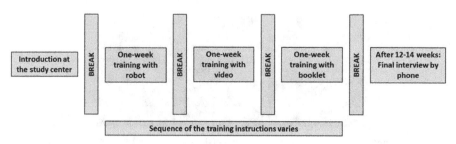

Fig. 3. Procedure of the study.

2.5 Analyses

To analyze the quantitative data from the questionnaires IBM SPSS 26 was used. The sample and questions were characterized with descriptive statistics (mean, standard deviation, frequencies). To compare the motivation to train with the robot at the introduction in the study center (T1) and after the training week with the humanoid robot (T2) the

Wilcoxon signed-rank test [35] was used, as non-parametric tests do not require a normal distribution of data and apply to small sample sizes.

The semi-structured telephone and face-to-face interviews (T2, T3) were recorded in writing, the statements were summarized and reported. No further qualitative content analysis [45] was performed due to the sample size and the explorative character of the study.

3 Results

3.1 Study Population

Eight older adults were recruited to participate. Due to acute physical impairment one participant was excluded. Five men and two women remained in the study population. Table 3 summarizes the characteristics of the study population.

Table 3. Characteristics of the study population.

	7 Participants
Age	74 (SD = 5.63, Range 67–84)
Nationality	Swiss
Canton	4 St.Gallen, 2 Thurgau, 1 Zurich
Residential area	5 more rural, 2 more urban
General state of health	1 excellent, 4 very good, 2 good
Activity per week	1 7-times, 1 6-times, 1 4-times, 1 3-times, 1 2-times, 2 1-time
Duration of activity	20 to 90 min
Activity in group or alone	3 in group, 3 both, 1 alone
Education	5 tertiary level education, 2 secondary level education
Household size	5 two-person household, 2 one-person household
Interested in technology	4 very interested, 3 interested
Contact with a robot before	2 at home, 1 at work, 1 somewhere else, 3 no contact before

3.2 Experiences of Older Adults Performing Exercises with the Robot at Home

All participants enjoyed the robot and they emphasized the joy in experiencing something new. They liked the humanoid appearance of the robot. Although there were some problems, all participants were able to exercise with the instruction of the socially assistive robot. But there were some difficulties that all participants had. From a technical point of view, there were five main difficulties. (1) When the participant started the robot, it took a very long time until the robot was ready for operation and the older adult could start with the training under the guidance of the robot. (2) The communication with the robot takes a long time because the robot was not ready to receive instructions or did not react immediately to instructions. (3) To receive instructions, the robot must recognize the face of a human being and then switch to "receive mode". However, the socially assistive robot used had problems recognizing the face of older adults and was therefore often not ready to receive instructions. This meant that the older adults had to bend down to the robot so that it could recognize them better. (4) The participants were instructed to put the robot on the floor because the robot was not very stable while demonstrating the exercises to the older adults. When the robot showed the exercises, it fell backward with six participants during at least one exercise. Partially it was able to stand up again on its own. (5) There were also acoustic problems, so the voice of the robot was perceived as an unpleasant computer voice, was not optimally understandable, and was sometimes perceived as strenuous.

3.3 Motivation

The humanoid looking socially assistive robot was experienced as motivating to be physically active. The training with the robot was judged as interesting and the exercises attractive. However, the participants could not rule out the possibility that over time, habituation effects may develop, and the robot may lose its attractiveness as a training coach. They often mentioned that they might lose interest in training with the robot over time. Due to the short training period of one week, this could not be verified. Also, the rigid instructions contribute to the decrease in the attractiveness of the robot as a training coach. For example, the instructions were often too long, were always repeated without variability, and therefore boring. In addition, there were too many and too long breaks (see Sect. 3.2), which unnecessarily lengthened the training program. Moreover, the older adults did not know whether the breaks were intended or whether the robot was defect.

The participants assessed the ability of the robot as a fitness coach with eight items. They were asked the questions after the instruction and first training with the robot at the study center (T1) and after the one-week training with the robot at home (T2). They could indicate their agreement from "1 = not at all" to "5 = very much". Table 4 shows the means and standard deviations. The Wilcoxon-tests show no significant results. So, there was no significant influence of the one-week training on the assessment of the robot as a training coach.

3.4 Comparison of the Three Types of Instructions

The video instruction was rated as good as the instruction by the robot. One participant found the video instruction better than the robot. Another participant preferred the robot because it is something new and therefore automatically has a certain attraction. Two participants pointed out that they have no space at home in front of their computer to exercise. One person found the video instructions more understandable. Other participants did not see a big difference between the video and the robot instructions. However, both the video and the robot instructions are experienced as more motivating than the written instructions. Whereby with the robot it is additionally mentioned that a relationship can be established with it. The written training instructions were rated worst. The

Table 4. Change in the self-developed assessment of the robot [58].

Question	T1 M (SD)	T2 M (SD)	Wilcoxon-test, exact significance, one-sided
How much did you enjoy training with NAO?	4.0 (0.82)	4.43 (0.98)	Z = −.828, p = .281, n = 7
Would you recommend NAO as a training coach to your friends?	2.17 (1.60)	2.50 (1.64)	Z = .000, p = .750, n = 6
How much would you like to train with NAO in the future?	3.14 (1.46)	2.29 (1.38)	Z = −1.857, P = .063, n = 7
Do you find NAO a good training coach?	3.43 (1.40)	2.71 (1.60)	Z = −1.089, p = .188, n = 7
How well could NAO motivate you for the training?	4.00 (1.41)	4.00 (1.73)	Z = −.378, p = .500, n = 7
Do you think NAO is more motivating than a human training coach?	1.43 (0.79)	1.29 (0.49)	Z = −1.000, p = .500, n = 7
Do you think NAO is more motivating than a training plan with video instructions?	3.57 (1.27)	2.57 (1.40)	Z = −1.382, p = .109, n = 7
Do you think NAO is more motivating than a written training plan?	4.71 (0.49)	3.57 (1.62)	Z = −1.857, p = .063, n = 7

T1: after introduction to robot training, T2: after one-week training with the robot, M: mean value, SD: standard deviation. 1 = not at all, 5 = very much

participants stated that they did not want to read while exercising. However, there are also individual exercises that are more comprehensible through the written instructions than just through the explanation of the robot.

The older adults would most likely wish to train together with a professional (sports teacher/therapist) who can give direct feedback, correct mistakes in the execution, and help in case of accidents, but this option was not offered in the study.

3.5 Recommendations

The study participants gave some recommendations on how to improve the training with the robot:

Features of the Robot: (1) The robot should be taller or elevated because it was rated to be too small. Since the robot was only allowed to be placed on the floor due to its instability, the older adults always had to bend down to communicate with the robot. (2) The communication with the robot should be easier. The participants did not want to wait to be recognized by the robot first. (3) It should be possible to adapt the sequence spontaneously by simple voice commands (e.g. "Stop", "Continue"). (4) The robot should not have any faults.

Other Desired Functions of the Robot: (1) The robot should have a reminder function integrated so that the participants can be reminded to train regularly. (2) Hearing aids should be compatible with the robot. (3) Breaks should be announced with their exact duration. (4) Feedback was required as to whether the exercises were being done correctly and the robot should correct incorrect movements.

Personalization: (1) Based on the feedback of the participating older adults, the training program of the robot should be individually adaptable and personalizable.

Variability: (1) The training program, but also the sentences, both in terms of content and structure, should have a greater variability to avoid boredom.

Environmental Factors: (1) The robot did not work on all floor coverings so environmental factors should be considered before implementation. For example, the robot worked worse on high carpets, but on smooth floors there was a risk that the robot would slip away.

Social Aspect: (1) Although the use of a robot as a training coach could motivate people to be physically active, the social aspect of the activities is just as important, especially for older adults, which is why a training group would be preferred.

4   Discussion

This study investigates whether a robot is motivating and practical for older people at home to perform physical exercises.

The study participants were well educated, interested in technology and four out of seven had previous experience with a robot. As only seven participants were included in the study, the sample is not representative. It was a highly selected study population which characteristics do not map the general population and therefore, results should not be generalized to other groups or the general population, although important points certainly apply in principle, and could be shown based on this group. The phenomenon that mainly well-educated seniors participate in studies about use of technology is known from other studies [e.g. 12, 73]. The number of participants who were interested in technology is in line with studies based on larger populations [e.g. 48, 72]. Regarding the percentage of people who already had experience with robots, findings for Germany values from 26% [26] and 27% [54] and for European countries 14% [14]. A recent survey showed 42% for Switzerland [41].

The participants emphasized that the experience with this new technical possibility was joyful. Also in the Technology Acceptance Model (TAM) 3 by Venkatesh and Bala [79] or in the Almere Model by Heerink, Kröse, Evers and Wielinga [34] "Perceived Enjoyment" is seen as a factor for the intention to use a technology. However, it should be considered that although the perceived enjoyment can influence acceptance, habituation effects should also be considered. It is known that after the novelty effect vanishes the interest in continuing to use the new technology decreases rapidly [57]. This circumstance could not be investigated in this study due to the short duration of the study. However, from the statements of the participants in the semi-structured interviews, it is clear that the robot's motivational factor quickly diminished when the novelty effect was exhausted and they doubt a long-term motivating effect, because already during the training week the always same and rigid exercises and instructions were perceived as not very entertaining.

The cute appearance of the robot was also positively highlighted. The positive evaluation of the humanoid appearance was mentioned, even if not specifically asked for it, also fits to the theory of the "uncanny valley" [50], according to which the acceptance of a robot increases the more human-like its appearance is. But there is a turning point where acceptance turns into rejection. A recent survey in Switzerland found that a quarter preferring a machine-like appearance and over a fifth preferring a human-like appearance [41]. Although the appearance was rated as cute, a larger robot was desired. This is mainly because the robot must recognize the face of the older adult to take orders. This could only be achieved if the older adult bent down toward the robot, which is probably why the wish for a larger robot was expressed.

The study clearly showed that technical defects, such as taking too long, not reacting, not recognizing, not being stable and acoustic problems, had a negative influence on the motivation to use the socially assistive robot. However, the participants did not rate these technical deficiencies of the robot as bad, because it was a well-educated sample with an affinity for technology, which was aware of the technical difficulties of new technologies, used to test technical systems and give critical feedback due to other studies at the institute. Differentiated feedback with error reports was not unusual for them.

The participants rated the socially assistive robot as motivating for physical activity, which gives a very positive image of this technical possibility. However, it should be considered that the participants only had the robot for one week during the study and had to train under its guidance three times. During this time, they were in a special test situation and were willing to comply with the study requirements. In addition, the study participants were already active before the training and perform sports exercises at least once a week. It is unclear how motivating the robot instruction can be over a longer period of several months and whether training would be carried out regularly. It is known that the acceptance of end users should be investigated over a longer period in their familiar environment in order to be able to make statements [40]. Even the non-significant differences in the assessment of the robot as a fitness coach are not surprising and should be repeated with a longer training period in between.

Improvements must be primarily of a technical nature, and here both features of the robot that need improvement and other desired functions of the robot have been mentioned several times. However, the individual adaptability and personalization are important too. Weidner, Redlich and Wulfsberg [84] do not see technical possibilities or economic considerations in the foreground for acceptance, but rather what is individually perceived as adequate. Also, Sankowski, Wollesen and Krause [59] indicate the optimal fit.

But also facilitating conditions from the Unified Theory of Acceptance and Use Technology (UTAUT) model [80] are discussed by noting in this concrete case that the robot does not work on all floor surfaces.

The study participants missed the social aspect of physical activity. Only one person carried out their previous physical activities alone, all other participants were used to being active in a group. So, on the one hand, it was mentioned that the supervision and control of the exercises were missing, but on the other hand, social control was missing. Social control is possible in the group so that even when people are living alone others would notice if they did not appear for training. A good application for a socially assistive robot would be the support of a human trainer. A human trainer should supervise the performance and assist, but the robot can motivate to be more active [10].

Overall, the participants found a socially assistive robot not useful for already active people, but for people who are not yet active. But they would not recommend the tested socially assistive robot mainly due to the technical problems and question of cost-benefit arises.

There are some limitations to the study that should be noted. The study was conducted as a real-life testing and therefore no lab conditions were present. There were technical problems of the robot and challenges to arrange personal appointments, so not all study participants went through the study in the same time span, and variation of the three conditions could not be balanced optimally. Since only one robot was available for all participants, it was not possible to test in parallel and the testing time had to be kept relatively short. However, the study was also conducted to get to know exactly these challenges in everyday life and what needs to be considered when using a socially assistive robot as a motivator for physical activity. Due to the short duration of the study, no long-term effects, no habituation effects and no effects on physical activity or other parameters such as the number of falls could be investigated. And no statement can be made whether the exercises would have been performed consistently over a longer period.

Furthermore, as already mentioned above, the study sample was not representative and even the meaningfulness of the mean value comparisons calculated is restricted because of the sample size.

An essential difference in the three conditions was that in the booklet and the video older adults showed the exercises. Furthermore, the influence of a reinforcer was not investigated, so in contrast to the written and video instructions, participants have been praised by the robot during the training.

5 Conclusions

The used socially assistive robot with a humanoid appearance was appreciated by the study participants and judged as motivating but not suitable because of its abilities and the strict sequence of the programmed movement exercises. Therefore, the older adults would not recommend this robot to their friends. It became clear, that this special robot is not suitable for autonomous exercise training for older adults at home. The study participants were highly motivated and interested in technology so it can be expected other less interested persons would rate the motivating effect less. Even if the study sample was small and explorative some factors from technology acceptance models like "perceived enjoyment", "facilitating conditions" or "social aspects" are mentioned, it became clear that they are important for further investigation. This research can help to try different ways to help older adults to be regularly active and to improve and adapt technical possibilities with the participation of older adults.

Acknowledgements. We thank all study participants and Zoe Brack, who programmed the robot as part of her master thesis.

References

1. Alzheimer's Disease International: World Alzheimer Report 2018. The state of the art of dementia research: New frontiers. Alzheimer's Disease International (ADI), London (2018). https://www.alz.co.uk/research/WorldAlzheimerReport2018.pdf
2. Bangsbo, J., Blackwell, J., Boraxbekk, C.-J., Caserotti, P., Dela, F., Evans, A.B., et al.: Copenhagen consensus statement 2019: physical activity and ageing. Br. J. Sports Med. **53**(14), 856–858 (2019). https://doi.org/10.1136/bjsports-2018-100451
3. Bedaf, S., Gelderblom, G.J., De Witte, L.: Overview and categorization of robots supporting independent living of elderly people: what activities do they support and how far have they developed. Assistive Technol.: Official J. RESNA **27**(2), 88–100 (2015). https://doi.org/10.1080/10400435.2014.978916
4. Beierlein, C., Kovaleva, A., Kemper, C., Rammstedt, B.: Ein Messinstrument zur Erfassung subjektiver Kompetenzerwartungen: Allgemeine Selbstwirksamkeit Kurzskala (ASKU). GESIS - Leibniz-Institut für Sozialwissenschaften, Mannheim (2012)
5. Bornschlegl, M., Fischer, R., Petermann, F.: Erfolgreiches kognitives Altern: Zusammenhang der kognitiven Leistungen mit Aktivität und Zufriedenheit. Zeitschrift für Neuropsychologie **27**, 173–187 (2016)
6. Brack, Z.: Programming and evaluating a robotic exercise coach to promote physical activity among elderly people. Master Thesis. ETH, Zurich (2019)
7. Broekens, J., Heerink, M., Rosendal, H.: Assistive social robots in elderly care: a review. Gerontechnology **8**, 2 (2009). https://doi.org/10.4017/gt.2009.08.02.002.00
8. Buhl, S.F., Beck, A.M., Christensen, B., Caserotti, P.: Effects of high-protein diet combined with exercise to counteract frailty in pre-frail and frail community-dwelling older adults: study protocol for a three-arm randomized controlled trial. Trials **21**(1), 637 (2020). https://doi.org/10.1186/s13063-020-04572-z
9. Büla, C., Jotterand, S., Martin, B.W., Bize, R., Lenoble-Hoskovec, C., Seematter-Bagnoud, L.: Bewegung im Alter: Dafür ist es nie zu spät! Swiss Med. Forum **14**, 836–841 (2014)
10. Čaić, M., Avelino, J., Mahr, D., Odekerken-Schröder, G., Bernardino, A.: Robotic versus human coaches for active aging: an automated social presence perspective. Int. J. Soc. Robot. **12**(4), 867–882 (2019). https://doi.org/10.1007/s12369-018-0507-2
11. Cunningham, C., O'Sullivan, R., Caserotti, P., Tully, M.A.: Consequences of physical inactivity in older adults: a systematic review of reviews and meta-analyses. Scand. J. Med. Sci. Sports **30**(5), 816–827 (2020). https://doi.org/10.1111/sms.13616
12. Dahms, R., Haesner, M.: Prävention und Gesundheitsförderung **13**(1), 46–52 (2017). https://doi.org/10.1007/s11553-017-0610-5
13. Dorner, T.E., Schindler, K.: Gesundheit im Alter: Selbständigkeit erhalten, Gebrechlichkeit vorbeugen. MANZ'sche Verlags- und Universitätsbuchhandlung GmbH, Wien (2017)
14. European Commission: Special Eurobarometer 460. Attitudes towards the impact of digitisation and automation on daily life (2017). https://ec.europa.eu/jrc/communities/sites/jrccties/files/ebs_460_en.pdf
15. European Commission: Bericht der Kommission an das europäische Parlament, den Rat, den europäischen Wirtschafts- und Sozialausschuss und den Ausschuss der Regionen über die Auswirkungen des demografischen Wandels. European Commission, Brüssel (2020)
16. European Commission: European Commission report on the impact of demographic change (2020). https://ec.europa.eu/info/sites/info/files/demography_report_2020.pdf

17. Eurostat: Population structure and ageing (2015). https://ec.europa.eu/eurostat/statistics-exp lained/index.php/Population_structure_and_ageing#Further_Eurostat_informationeuropa. eu/public_opinion/archives/ebs/ebs_382_en.pdf

18. Fasola, J., Matarić, M.J.: Comparing physical and virtual embodiment in a socially assistive robot exercise coach for the elderly. Center for Robotics and Embedded Systems, Los Angeles (2011)

19. Fasola, J., Matarić, M.J.: Using socially assistive human–robot interaction to motivate physical exercise for older adults. Proc. IEEE **100**(8), 2512–2526 (2012)

20. Fasola, J., Matarić, M.J.: A socially assistive robot exercise coach for the elderly. J. Hum. Robot Interaction **2**(2), 3–32 (2013)

21. Federal Agency for Civic Education [bpb]: Altersstruktur und Bevölkerungsentwicklung (2018). https://www.bpb.de/nachschlagen/zahlen-und-fakten/europa/70503/altersstruktur#: ~:text=Bezogen%20auf%20die%2028%20Staaten,auf%2028%2C5%20Prozent%20erh% C3%B6hen. Accessed 09 Aug 2020

22. Federal Statistical Office: Grad der Einschränkung in den Alltagsaktivitäten (ADL) (2019). https://www.bfs.admin.ch/bfs/de/home/statistiken/kataloge-datenbanken/grafiken.assetd etail.8066066.html. Accessed 23 Jul 2020

23. Federal Statistical Office: Grad der Einschränkung in den instrumentellen Alltagsaktivitäten (IADL) (2019). https://www.bfs.admin.ch/bfs/de/home/statistiken/gesundheit/gesundheitsz ustand/alter.assetdetail.8066068.html. Accessed 23 Jul 2020

24. Federal Statistical Office: Künftige Bevölkerungsentwicklung der Schweiz und der Kantone 2020–2050. Neuchâtel: Bundesamt für Statistik, Neuchâtel (2020)

25. Flandorfer, P.: Population ageing and socially assistive robots for elderly persons: the importance of sociodemographic factors for user acceptance. Int. J. Popul. Res. 829835 (2012). https://doi.org/10.1155/2012/829835

26. Forsa. Politik- und Sozialforschung GmbH: Service-Robotik: Mensch-Technik-Interaktion im Alltag. Ergebnisse einer repräsentativen Befragung. Berlin (2016). https://www.bmbf.de/ files/BMBF_forsa_Robotik_FINAL2016.pdf

27. Füzéki, E., Banzer, W.: Bewegung und Gesundheit im Alter. In: Banzer, W. (ed.) Körperliche Aktivität und Gesundheit, pp. 139–155. Springer, Heidelberg (2017). https://doi.org/10.1007/ 978-3-662-50335-5_10

28. Gadde, P., Kharrazi, H., Patel, H., MacDorman, K.F.: Toward monitoring and increasing exercise adherence in older adults by robotic intervention: a proof of concept study. J. Robot. (2011). https://doi.org/10.1155/2011/438514

29. Gschwind, Y.J., Pfenninger, B.: Training zur Sturzprävention. Bfu-Fachdokumentation 2.104. Beratungsstelle für Unfallverhütung, Bern (2016)

30. Guneysu Ozgur, A., et al.: Gamified motor training with tangible robots in older adults: a feasibility study and comparison with the young. Front. Aging Neurosci. **12**, 59 (2020). https://doi.org/10.3389/fnagi.2020.00059

31. Gunzelmann, T., Brähler, C., Hessel, A., Brähler, E.: Körpererleben im Alter. Zeitschrift für Gerontopsychologie -psychiatrie **12**(1), 40–54 (1999)

32. Haigh, E.A.P., Bogucki, O.E., Sigmon, S.T., Blazer, D.G.: Depression among older adults: a 20-year update on five common myths and misconceptions. Am. J. Geriatr. Psychiatry. **26**(1), 107–122 (2018). https://doi.org/10.1016/j.jagp.2017.06.011

33. Hedtke-Becker, A., Hoevels, R., Otto, U., Stumpp, G., Beck, S.: Zu Hause wohnen wollen bis zuletzt. In: Pohlmann, S. (ed.) Altern mit Zukunft, pp. 141–176, Springer, Wiesbaden (2012). https://doi.org/10.1007/978-3-531-19418-9_6

34. Heerink, M., Kröse, B., Evers, V., Wielinga, B.: Assessing acceptance of assistive social agent technology by older adults: the almere model. Int. J. Social Robot. **2**(4), 361–375 (2010). https://doi.org/10.1007/s12369-010-0068-5

35. Higgins, J.J.: An Introduction to Modern Nonparametric Statistics. Brooks/Cole, Pacific Grove (2004)
36. International Federation of Robotics: Service robots (2020). https://ifr.org/service-robots/. Accessed 23 Jun 2020
37. Kashi, S., Levy-Tzedek, S.: Smooth leader or sharp follower? Playing the mirror game with a robot. Restor. Neurol. Neurosci. **36**(2), 147–159 (2018)
38. Krug, S., Jordan, S., Mensink, G.B.M., Müters, S., Finger, J.D., Lampert, T.: Körperliche Aktivität. Ergebnisse der Studie zur Gesundheit Erwachsener in Deutschland (DEGS1). Bundesgesundheitsblatt **56**, 765–771 (2013)
39. Lebedeva, A., Steinert, A., Buchem, I., Merceron, A., Kreutel, J., Haesner, M.: Trainingskonzepte seniorengerecht und motivational entwickeln – Handlungsempfehlungen aus Wissenschaft und Praxis, vol. 8. AAL-Kongress, Frankfurt am Main (2015)
40. Lehmann, S., Hämmerle, V., Pauli, C., Misoch, S.: Partizipative Testung assistiver Technik. Das Konzept der Living Labs 65+ des IKOA-FHS. In: Friedrich, P., Fuchs, D. (eds.) 6. Ambient Medicine Forum. Assistive Technik für selbstbestimmtes Wohnen, pp. 103–107, Cuvillier, Göttingen (2019)
41. Lehmann, S., Ruf, E., Misoch, S.: Robot use for older adults – attitudes, wishes and concerns. first results from Switzerland. In: Stephanidis, C., Antona, M. (eds.) HCII 2020. CCIS, vol. 1226, pp. 64–70. Springer, Cham (2020). https://doi.org/10.1007/978-3-030-50732-9_9
42. Löllgen, H., Leyk, D.: Prävention durch Bewegung. Bedeutung der körperlichen Leistungsfähigkeit. Der Internist **53**(6), 663–670 (2012)
43. Marek, K.D., Rantz, M.J.: Ageing in place: a new model for long-term care. Nurs. Adm. Q. **24**(3), 1–11 (2000)
44. Martinez-Martin, E., Costa, A., Cazorla, M.: PHAROS 2.0-A PHysical Assistant RObot system improved. Sensors (Basel, Switz.) **19**(20), 4531 (2019). https://doi.org/10.3390/s19204531
45. Mayring, P.: Qualitative content analysis. Forum Qualitative Sozialforschung / Forum Qual. Soc. Res. 1(2), Art. 20 (2000)
46. Mercay, C., Burla, L., Widmer, M.: Gesundheitspersonal in der Schweiz. Bestandesaufnahme und Prognosen bis 2030 (Obsan Bericht 71). Schweizerisches Gesundheitsobservatorium, Neuchâtel (2016)
47. Mercay, C., Grünig, A.: Gesundheitspersonal in der Schweiz – Zükünftiger Bedarf bis 2030 und die Folgen für den Nachwuchsbedarf (Obsan Bulletin 12/2016). Schweizerisches Gesundheitsobservatorium, Neuchâtel (2016)
48. Mies, C.: Akzeptanz von Smart Home Technologien: Einfluss von subjektivem Pflegebedarf und Technikerfahrung bei älteren Menschen. Untersuchung im Rahmen des Projekts «Accepting Smart Homes». Diplomarbeit, Wien (2011)
49. Misoch, S.: Qualitative Interviews. 2., erweiterte und aktualisierte Auflage. De Gruyter Oldenbourg, Berlin (2019)
50. Mori, M.: The uncanny valley. Energy **7**, 33–35 (1970)
51. Mura, G.: Physical activity in depressed elderly. a systematic review. Clin. Pract. Epidemiol. Ment. Health **9**, 125–135 (2013). https://doi.org/10.2174/1745017901309010125
52. Müller, C., Lautenschläger, S., Voigt-Radloff, S.: Potential analysis for research on occupational therapy-led physical exercise programmes and home environment adaptation programmes to prevent falls for elderly people living at home. Int. J. Health Professions **3**, 85–106 (2016)
53. Ng, T.P.: Old age depression: worse clinical course, brighter treatment prospects? Lancet Psychiatry **5**(7), 533–534 (2018). https://doi.org/10.1016/S2215-0366(18)30186-X
54. Nitto, H., Taniyama, D., Inagaki, H.: Social acceptance and impact of robots and artificial intelligence. Findings of survey in Japan, the U.S. and Germany. Nomura Research Institute

(NRI Papers, 211) (2017). https://www.nri.com/-/media/Corporate/en/Files/PDF/knowle dge/report/cc/papers/2017/np2017211.pdf?la=en&hash=A730998FD55F6D58DF95F347 9E3B709FC8EF83F4. Accessed 23 Jun 2020

55. Pilotto, A., Boi, R., Petermans, J.: Technology in geriatrics. Age Ageing **47**(6), 771–774 (2018). https://doi.org/10.1093/ageing/afy026

56. Pro Senectute Homepage. https://www.prosenectute.ch. Accessed 06 Aug 2020

57. Rosenthal-von der Pütten, A.M., et al.: Investigations on empathy towards humans and robots using fMRI. Comput. Hum. Behav. **33**, 201–212 (2014)

58. Ruf, E., Lehmann, S., Misoch, S.: Motivating older adults to exercise at home: suitability of a humanoid robot. In: Guldemond, N., Ziefle, M., Maciaszek, L. (eds.) Proceedings of the 6th International Conference on Information and Communication Technologies for Ageing Well and e-Health, pp. 113–120 (2020). https://doi.org/10.5220/0009341001130120

59. Sankowski, O., Wollesen, B., Krause, D.: Ein methodischer Ansatz für die Entwicklung angepasster und altersgerechter Produkte am Beispiel einer Aufstehhilfe. In: Weidner, R., Redlich, T. (eds.) Erste Transdisziplinäre Konferenz zum Thema Technische Unter-stützungssysteme, die die Menschen wirklich wollen, pp 66–77. Helmut-Schmidt-Universität, Hamburg (2014)

60. Satariano, W.A., Guralnik, J.M., Jackson, R.J., Marottoli, R.A., Phelan, E.A., Prohaska, T.R.: Mobility and aging: new directions for public health action. Am. J. Public Health **102**(8), 1508–1515 (2012). https://doi.org/10.2105/AJPH.2011.300631

61. Schaakxs, R., Comijs, H.C., Lamers, F., Kok, R.M., Beekman, A.T.F., Penninx, B.W.J.H.: Associations between age and the course of major depressive disorder: a 2-year longitudinal cohort study. Lancet Psychiatry **5**(7), 581–590 (2018). https://doi.org/10.1016/S2215-036 6(18)30166-4

62. Schneider, S., Kümmert, F.: Exercising with a humanoid companion is more effective than exercising alone. In: 16th IEEE International Conference on Humanoid Robots, pp. 495–501 (2016)

63. Scholes, S., Mindell, J.: Physical activity in adults. Health Surv. Engl. **1**(2), 1–49 (2012)

64. Schuch, F.B., et al.: Physical activity protects from incident anxiety: a meta-analysis of prospective cohort studies. Depression Anxiety **36**(9), 846–858 (2019). https://doi.org/10. 1002/da.22915

65. Schuch, F.B., et al.: Physical activity and incident depression: a meta-analysis of prospective cohort studies. Am. J. Psychiatry **175**(7), 631–648 (2018). https://doi.org/10.1176/appi.ajp. 2018.17111194

66. Schulz, R., Wahl, H.-W., Matthews, J.T., De Vito Dabbs, A., Beach, S.R., Czaja, S.J.: Advancing the aging and technology agenda in gerontology. Gerontologist **55**(5), 724–734 (2015). https://doi.org/10.1093/geront/gnu071

67. Seifert, A., Meidert, U.: Quantified seniors. Prävention und Gesundheitsförderung **13**, 353–360 (2018)

68. Senderovich, H., Tsai, P.M.: Do exercises prevent falls among older adults: Where are we now? A systematic review. J. Am. Med. Directors Assoc. Advance online publication (2020). https://doi.org/10.1016/j.jamda.2020.05.010

69. Shen, Z., Wu, Y.: Investigation of practical use of humanoid robots in elderly care centres. In: Proceedings of the 4th International Conference on Human Agent Interaction, pp. 63–66 (2016)

70. Sherrington, C., et al.: Exercise to prevent falls in older adults: An updated systematic review and meta-analysis. Br. J. Sports Med. **51**, 1750–1758 (2016)

71. Sicher stehen – sicher gehen Homepage. https://www.sichergehen.ch. Accessed 06 Aug 2020

72. Stadelhofer, C.: Möglichkeiten und Chancen der Internetnutzung durch Ältere. Zeitschrift für Gerontologie und Geriatrie **33**, 186–194 (2000)

73. Steinert, A., Haesner, M., Tetley, A., Steinhagen-Thiessen, E.: Nutzungsverhalten einer Gesundheitsapplikation zum Selbstmonitoring von Senioren. Prävention und Gesundheitsförderung **10**(4), 281–286 (2015). https://doi.org/10.1007/s11553-015-0510-5

74. Sun, F., Norman, I.J., While, A.E.: Physical activity in older people: a systematic review. BMC Public Health **13**, 449 (2013). https://doi.org/10.1186/1471-2458-13-449

75. Torta, E., Oberzaucher, J., Werner, F., Cuijpers, R.H., Juola, J.F.: Attitudes towards socially assistive robots in intelligent homes: results from laboratory studies and field trials. J. Hum.-Robot Interaction **1**(2), 76–99 (2013)

76. Tully, M.A., et al.: Sedentary behaviour, physical activity and mental health in older adults: an isotemporal substitution model. Scand. J. Med. Sci. Sports, Advance online publication (2020). https://doi.org/10.1111/sms.13762

77. Vancea, M., Solé-Casals, J.: Population aging in the European information societies: towards a comprehensive research agenda in eHealth innovations for elderly. Aging Dis. **7**(4), 526–539 (2015). https://doi.org/10.14336/AD.2015.1214

78. Vaupel, J.: Setting the stage: a generation of centenarians? Washington Q. **23**(3), 197–200 (2000)

79. Venkatesh, V., Bala, H.: Technology acceptance model 3 and a research agenda on interventions. Decis. Sci. **39**(2), 273–315 (2008)

80. Venkatesh, V., Morris, M.G., Davis, G.B., Davis, F.D.: User acceptance of information technology: toward a unified view. Manag. Inf. Syst. Q. **27**(3), 425–478 (2003)

81. Voelcker-Rehage, C., Godde, B., Staudinger, U.M.: Bewegung, körperliche und geistige Mobilität im Alter. Gesundheitsschutz **49**, 558–566 (2006)

82. Ware, J.E.: SF-36 health survey update. Spine **25**, 3130–3139 (2000)

83. Weber, D., et al.: Gesundheit und Lebensqualität im Alter. Grundlagen für kantonale Aktionsprogramme «Gesundheitsförderung im Alter» (Bericht 5). Gesundheitsförderung Schweiz, Bern (2016)

84. Weidner, R., Redlich, T., Wulfsberg, J.P.: Technik, die die Menschn wollen. Unterstützungssysteme für Beruf und Alltag. In: Weidner, R., Redlich, T. (eds.) Erste Transdisziplinäre Konferenz zum Thema "Technische Unterstützungssysteme, die die Menschen wirklich wollen", pp. 1–8, Helmut-Schmidt-Universität, Hamburg (2014)

85. Werner, F., Krainer, D., Oberzaucher, J., Werner, K.: Evaluation of the acceptance of a social assistive robot for physical training support together with older users and domain experts. Assistive Technol.: From Res. Pract.: AAATE **33**, 137–142 (2013). https://doi.org/10.3233/978-1-61499-304-9-137

86. Werner, F., Werner, K., Oberzaucher, J.: Evaluation of the acceptance of a socially assistive robot by older users within the project KSERA. In: Proceedings: Lebensqualität im Wandel von Demografie und Technik. Deutscher AAL-Kongress (2013)

87. World Health Organization.: World report on disability (2011). https://www.who.int/disabilities/world_report/2011/report.pdf

88. World Health Organization: Global action plan for the prevention and control of noncommunicable diseases 2013–2020 (2013). https://apps.who.int/iris/bitstream/handle/10665/94384/9789241506236_eng.pdf

89. World Health Organization.: World report on ageing and health. World Health Organization, Geneva (2015)

90. World Health Organization.: Management of physical health conditions in adults with severe mental disorders. WHO Guidelines (2018). https://apps.who.int/iris/bitstream/handle/10665/275718/9789241550383-eng.pdf

91. Wullems, J.A., Verschueren, S.M.P., Degens, H., Morse, C.I., Onambélé, G.L.: A review of the assessment and prevalence of sedentarism in older adults, its physiology/health impact and non-exercise mobility counter-measures. Biogerontology **17**(3), 547–565 (2016). https://doi.org/10.1007/s10522-016-9640-1

Comparison of Video and Radar Contactless Heart Rate Measurements

Linda Senigagliesi⬡, Manola Ricciuti$^{(\boxtimes)}$⬡, Gianluca Ciattaglia⬡, Adelmo De Santis⬡, and Ennio Gambi⬡

Università Politecnica delle Marche, 60131 Ancona, Italy
{l.senigagliesi,adelmo.desantis,e.gambi}@univpm.it,
{m.ricciuti,g.ciattaglia}@pm.univpm.it

Abstract. One of the most relevant aspects investigated by the scientific community in the healthcare field is the detection of vital parameters, such as the heart rate, through the use of contactless technologies, often considered more comfortable and unobtrusive for the subjects in exam. In particular, the main goal is to develop real-time oriented algorithms able to minimize the errors and to obtain results as close as possible to those achieved by clinical instruments, especially with the aim of carrying out a constant home monitoring for the elderly. In this paper two contactless methodologies for the heart rate estimation are analyzed, exploiting different approaches. In the first we first apply face recognition methods on RGB videos, and we then use well known algorithms for the extraction of the heart rate, such as Eulerian Video Magnification, Independent Component Analysis, Principal Component Analysis and Skin Detection. In the second the cardiac frequency is extracted through a mmWave radar by applying two multiple-input multiple-output (MIMO) algorithms, one based on the Fast Fourier Transform (FFT) and one on the MUltiple SIgnal Classification (MUSIC) algorithm. For both approaches, the results are compared to those obtained using more standard instruments, such as a pulse oximeter, proving the accuracy and precision of the implemented systems.

Keywords: Contactless sensor · Heart rate · mmWave radar

1 Introduction

One of the new technological frontiers in the healthcare field is that of the detection of vital parameters such as the heart rate (HR) and the heart rate variability (HRV) through the use of remote technologies. Conventional clinical equipment available today for heart rate monitoring is in most cases expensive and difficult to place. The electrocardiograph, for example, requires a considerable number of electrodes and cables which, besides being inconvenient in certain cases of clinical analysis, must be positioned on the body of the patient by trained personnel.

Supported by Università Politecnica delle Marche.

M. Ziefle et al. (Eds.): ICT4AWE 2020, CCIS 1387, pp. 96–113, 2021.
https://doi.org/10.1007/978-3-030-70807-8_6

New contactless technologies for the remote monitoring of vital parameters have emerged in the last years as a valid alternative to classical standard methodologies. Among these, particular interest is gained by methodologies based on radar and video processing. Recently, progresses have been made in the design of algorithms capable of extracting vital parameters from the analysis of video signals. Among them, Eulerian Video Magnification (EVM) [30] and Independent Component Analysis (ICA) proved to achieve good results, placing themselves as an efficient alternative to well-validated and traditionally used methods. Another considered method in this field is the principal component analysis (PCA), a technique deriving from linear algebra studies which is widely used in the most varied areas and consists in selecting only the main components a huge amount of data.

In this paper, we study and compare different contactless techniques to estimate the HR. With respect to [24], we consider alternative solutions for radar and video processing in order to improve results and reduce the computational burden of the algorithms. We first study the application of the ICA+PCA algorithm on the video signal, showing that it contributes to decrease the computational cost at the expenses of a growing number of detection errors. To overcome this issue we introduce the use of the skin detection technique, which allows to achieve a good trade-off between accuracy and low computational cost, could represent a valid solution to design an automatic mechanism for the HR measurement. As regards the radar processing, we apply the MUltiple SIgnal Classification (MUSIC) algorithm as an alternative to the more classic Fast Fourier Transform (FFT) to improve the detection of the correct peaks on the spectrum, from those we derive the value of the HR. In order to estimate their accuracy of the mentioned methods, we compare the results obtained with those measured with more standard and provably precise technologies, such as a pulse oximeter, proving that we are able to obtain a very small error even using contactless methodologies and low cost devices.

2   Related Work

In the last years several methods to extract HR and other vital parameters, such as the HRV and the cardiac frequency, have been proposed in literature, mainly based on the analysis of photoplethysmography (PPG) and videoplethysmography (VPG) signals. The most studied algorithms are those that exploit the EVM method or the Independent Component Analysis (ICA). In [9] the heart rate is derived through EVM algorithm using a Microsoft Kinect v2 device, proving that the resulting error is negligible and can be further improved by knowing the life style of the analysed subject. Similarly, in [26] the VPG is obtained using the ICA method, with the purpose of measuring the blood pressure through the analysis of the Pulse Transit Time (PPT) derived from the VPG signal.

Also in [21] the ICA method is used not only to obtain the HR, but also the HRV and the respiratory frequency, with good results for all the vital parameters. In particular, the Joint Approximate Diagonalization of Eigenmatrices (JADE)

ICA method is considered, by selecting the principal component having the maximum peak in frequency. Once measured the VPG signal, peaks and RR intervals (where RR identifies the intervals between successive heartbeats, i.e. the distance between two consecutive R waves) are determined and the HRV and the respiratory frequency are derived from the tachogram.

ICA and EVM methods are compared in [1] by considering results of both methods for the HRV extraction. It is proved that the ICA has a better performance since the EVM shows a high level of noise at the high frequencies in the power spectrum of the tachogram.

The PCA method, before being used to derive the VPG signal through the analysis of video signals, has been applied directly to the PPG signal obtained from an oximeter to determine the vital parameters. In [16] PCA of a PPG signal is used to determine the respiratory frequency. The intensity variation of the PPG signal due to respiration is visible in the coefficients of the principal components. In [17] it is proved that, besides respiratory frequency, also cardiac frequency can be derived by applying the Ensemble Empirical Mode Decomposition (EEMD) on the signal, thus obtaining a certain number of Intrinsic Mode Functions (IMF). The IMF subjected to artifacts (noise) are then eliminated thanks to a spectral analysis and the PCA is then applied on the remaining IMF. Finally, after selecting the first main component containing information on cardiac activity, the frequency attributable to the cardiac frequency is obtained from the latter spectrum.

Another possible application of PCA and, in particular, of multiscale PCA on the PPG signal considers the use of principal components to remove both voluntary and involuntary movement artifacts, as shown in [22], where it is also proved that PCA achieves an accuracy similar to that achieved by ICA. Several papers describe the differences between ICA and PCA methods. In [8] detection, face tracking and skin detection techniques are compared, also making a comparison between the various ICA techniques (JADE ICA, FAST ICA, KERNEL ICA, Second Order Blind Identification) and PCA, showing that PCA has a lower mean square error compared to various ICA methods. An example of the use of the ICA and PCA method on all three channels on RGB video for the determination of the VPG signal is given in [13]. Two different approaches are used in this work: in the first one the whole face is considered, while in the second only the region of interest (ROI) representing the individual's forehead is taken into consideration. The results obtained show that the analysis of the forehead has an accuracy similar to the analysis of the entire face.

Attempts to use other image formats outside of RGB have been made in [25], arguing that the limit of the PCA, like that of the ICA, is the fact that it is not possible to know a priori which channel to use, and showing that it is also possible to derive HR by analyzing YUV images. In fact, it is shown that from a spectral point of view the VPG signals obtained from the analysis of the components Y, U, V are very similar to the VPG signals obtained by using the two ICA and PCA methods on the three channels R, G, B. This correlation is demonstrated by the linear dependence between the two color spaces.

As regards the extraction of HRV from PPG signal, authors of [2] consider the analysis of the PPG signal measured with a pulseoximeter. After determining the R peaks, the LF/HF ratio is derived from the power spectrum of the previously obtained tachogram. In [19] the led light and the camera in a smartphone are used. The subjects involved in the experiments were simply asked to place their finger on the camera and on the LED of the smart phone. To obtain the PPG signal, authors propose to select a ROI of the size of 80 × 80 pixels and to average the intensity of the red channel, whose variations are due to blood flow. The results confirm that the difference between the HRV assessment obtained through the ECG or through the proposed method is minimal. In [7] video acquisitions were made through a smart phone and in different light conditions. The HR was obtained with the ICA method and others such as the Canonical Components Analysis (CCA) method, the CHRXMY and CHRXOY method, which are based on the study of the signal chrominance obtained through linear combinations of the RGB channels, and, finally, the Pulse Blood Volume (PBV) method. Then, by comparing the results in relation to the level and type of light, it was demonstrated that the ICA method is, together with the CCA method, the one that gave the best results.

The purpose of the work in [14] is to extract the heart rate n variable light conditions and non-rigid movements of the subject. After using the Discriminative Response Map Fitting (DRMF) method to generate a ROI mask on the first frame and after implementing the Kanade-Lucas-Tomasi (KLT) algorithm for face tracking, the raw VPG signal is constructed by applying a spatial average on the green channel of the ROI. The authors propose to obtain an estimate of the interfering variations on the green channel by exploiting the Distance Regularized Level Set Evolution (DRLSE) method applied on the background of the frame. In this way, the intensity variations on the green channel in the background can be considered unrelated to the useful signal. Finally, to remove movement artifacts, the VPG signal is divided into segments which are subjected to a series of filters to eliminate the signal out of the useful bandwidth.

Radar systems proved their effectiveness in many scenarios different from the one they were originally designed for. Recently, these systems have attracted the attention of the medical field, thanks to their ability to provide high precision measurements at a reduced cost. In particular, a special interest has raised about the remote monitoring of vital parameters [20]. In [15,28] vital signs are extracted by using a Continuous Wave (CW) radar, while the same analysis is performed through an impulsive Ultra wideband (UWB) radar in [23] and a Frequency-Modulated Continuous-Wave (FMCW) radar in [18,27]. The operational frequency of this kind of radar is in the range 24–80 GHz [4]; the use of such high frequencies allows measurements with good resolution, thus making it possible to analyze variations in very small displacements, such as those produced by the heartbeat.

The rest of the paper is organized as follows. In Sect. 3 we describe the algorithm developed for the extraction of the HR from the video signal processing, along with the ICA+PCA method and the skin detection. The radar signal processing and the MUSIC algorithm are presented in Sect. 4. Section 5 contains the results obtained and the comparison between the considered measurement techniques. Final considerations and remarks are provided in Sect. 6.

3   Heart Rate Estimation from Video

In this section we describe the techniques and algorithms applied for HR extraction through the video processing of a subject's face, starting from the EVM method [30]. This technique exploits the slight variations in the skin color, generated by the blood flow in the tissues, and amplifies them. The entire algorithm is briefly presented in Figs. 1, 2.

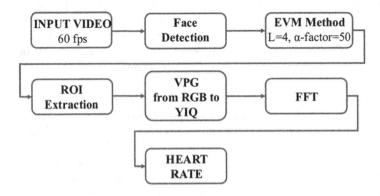

Fig. 1. Main scheme of the video signal processing algorithm.

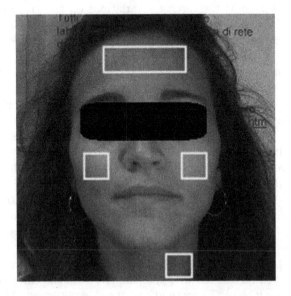

Fig. 2. Region of interest (ROI) selection on a subject's face.

The EVM method allows to amplify the skin color starting from the RGB images acquired on the faces of the subjects under test. RGB images captured from video are first transformed into YIQ, a color space made up of luminance components Y and chrominance and quadrature IQ. For the elaborations, a color amplification factor α equal 50 is considered, in order to choose a value that does not distort the color after the EVM processing. The α factor depends on the light of the environment where the images are acquired. A series of temporal and spatial filters are then applied to decompose the images by subsampling them until they have a resolution that is 2^L times lower than the original ones, where L is the considered level. The final resolution of the images, which include only the faces, has a dimension which varies from 300×300 to 18×18 pixels. The next step is the selection on the face of the ROIs from which extract to heart rate, corresponding to the forehead, the cheeks and the neck. The ROIs selection allows both to reduce the computational burden and to avoid the selection of useless parts of the image, such as the background behind the face.

In order to extract the trend of the signal over time, we select the luminance component from the ROIs, thus obtaining the VPG signal over time. It highlights the presence of peaks from those we can derive the heart rate, converting the signal from the time domain to frequency through the Fast Fourier Transform (FTT). The bandwidth of interest of the selected frequencies goes from 50 to 120 bpm (i.e. from 0.83 2 Hz), considering standard values of subjects at rest.

3.1   ICA+PCA Method

The ICA method is used to decompose the initial RGB channels into separate channels to treat them independently, as shown in Fig. 3. Empirically, it is observed that the best results are obtained with the green channel, so this will be selected in the following.

ICA method is based on the assumption that the observed data x can be represented as the linear combination of signals s produced by single underlying sources, or, in formulas

$$x = \mathbf{A}s, \tag{1}$$

where A is the *mixing matrix*, a squared and invertible matrix which, by mixing the signals s through the matrix product, reproduces our observed data x. The core of ICA method is therefore to estimate $\mathbf{A}^{-1}$ in order to recover s by inverting (1).

For this approach we consider the same ROIs selected as for the EVM method.

After having selected the green channel, the elaboration is performed through the PCA technique, in order to avoid the manual selection of the ROIs and to consider the principal components related to the higher intensity of the signal. The process is therefore automatised to speed up the entire process, thus allowing real time elaborations (Fig. 4).

To implement this approach we rely on the Singular Value Decomposition (SVD) technique, which consists in the decomposition of an $\mathbf{X}$ matrix of any size

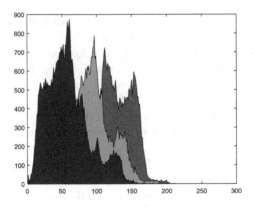

Fig. 3. RGB image histogram.

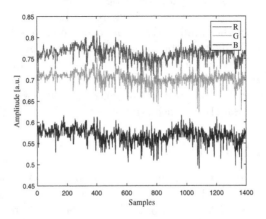

Fig. 4. ICA for RGB channels, choice of the green channel G. (Color figure online)

into the product of other matrices which, given their properties, can simplify subsequent calculations involving $\mathbf{X}$. If a $\mathbf{X}$ is a real matrix, we can decompose it into three matrices

$$\mathbf{X} = \mathbf{U}\mathbf{\Sigma}\mathbf{V}^{-1}. \tag{2}$$

The diagonal values of $\mathbf{\Sigma}$ are known as "singular values" of the matrix $\mathbf{X}$, while the columns of $\mathbf{U}$ are known as "left singular vectors" of $\mathbf{X}$ and the columns of $\mathbf{V}$ are the "right singular vectors of $\mathbf{X}$. By projecting the data on the principal axes we obtain the principal components given by

$$\mathbf{X}\mathbf{V} = \mathbf{U}\mathbf{\Sigma}\mathbf{V}^{T}\mathbf{V} = \mathbf{U}\mathbf{\Sigma}, \tag{3}$$

which, once derived $\mathbf{U}$ and $\mathbf{\Sigma}$ from the SVD, can be easily computed.

The use of PCA avoids the ROIs selection, considering instead the 100 principal eigenvalues of the diagonal matrix $\mathbf{\Sigma}$, which are those useful to extract the features of interest, i.e. those related to the heart rate. The principal components provide the greater intensity of the signal extracted from the green channel.

However, PCA leads to a greater error, which can be reduced by introducing the skin detection technique, as described in the next section.

With respect to the EVM described in Sect. 3, the ICA+PCA method has a lower computational cost, which allows a higher computation speed. Moreover, there is no need of a manual setting of the face regions to be analyzed to extract the heartbeat, since only the pixels with higher intensity are chosen, together with the principal coefficients related to these intensity values. However, with ICA+PCA the number of detection errors increases, but it could represent the ideal trade-off between the choice of an automatic and real-time oriented mechanism and the accuracy of results.

3.2   Skin Detection

In order to reduce the comparison error with the reference method (pulse oximeter) but still maintain an automatic mechanism, the tests are processed with ICA+PCA in addition with the Skin Detection. This technique allows to identify a macro region of the face to extract the heart beat, without recurring to the ROIs selection. The choice of the principal components is strengthened by Skin Detection. By implementing this method the presence of the skin is recognized from digital images of subjects.

The scheme of the algorithm is depicted in Fig. 5. It goes through five main steps for each frame:

1. *Transformation of the Color Space from RGB to YCbCr*: Y is luminance component and Cb and Cr are the chrominance components blue-difference and red-difference, as shown in Fig. 6. Through the color space YCbCr the primary colors corresponding approximately to red, green and blue are elaborated into perceptually significant information. Y is in the range [16/255, 235/255], Cb and Cr are in the range [16/255, 240/255].
2. *Setting of the Thresholds for the Chrominance Components*: The thresholds for chrominance levels are set in such a way as to surely enclose the values corresponding, in this case, to the subjects' faces, excluding the background of the image. After having evaluated them empirically, it resulted that the same values are suitable to any subject among those analyzed in the dataset. The values are the following:
   - $0.40 \leq Cb \leq 0.46$;
   - $0.56 \leq Cr \leq 0.61$.
3. *Creation of a Binary Mask to Distinguish the Pixels Corresponding to the Skin from the Others*: All the pixels of the examined image are made binary by imposing a mask that sets to 1 the pixels in the defined chrominance range, leaving the others to 0.
4. *Filling of any "holes" within the Macro-region (Agglomeration of Large Area Pixels) Detected and Corresponding to the Presence of Skin*: The small "holes" are filled and the macro-regions with an area of at least 1000 pixels are considered for the subsequent heart rate estimate processing.
5. *Finding the Box Containing the Face*: Finally, a rectangular bounding-box is built to identify the region to be considered for the extraction of the heartbeat. In this case, it can be observed that the neck is excluded from processing.

An example of the application of the different steps of the algorithm on images is shown in Fig. 7.

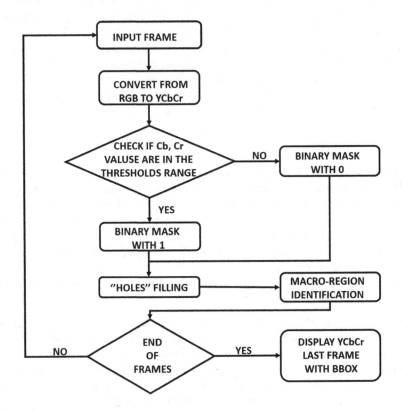

Fig. 5. Skin Detection algorithm.

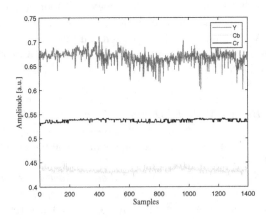

Fig. 6. YCbCr map.

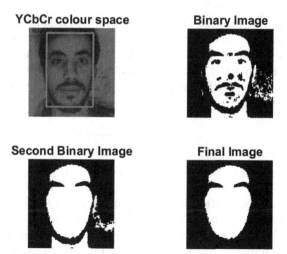

Fig. 7. Example of application of the algorithm.

4 Heart Rate Estimation from Radar

The use of radar systems to determine the physiological parameters of a subject is implemented with the application of a technology that comes from the automotive world. Automotive radars are in fact capable of achieving extremely high precision at reduced costs. In our tests we exploit the AWR1843 radar provided by Texas Instruments [10], a Multiple-Input Multiple-Output (MIMO) radar with a fully integrated system containing a RF section, a DSP processor, an analog-to-digital converter (ADC) and a micro-controller; 4 receivers and 3 transmitters are available. A scheme of the device is reported in Fig. 8.

A high precision in the definition of the target position is needed for the subject's HR detection, since, as described in the following, the heart activity is studied through the analysis of the phase of the signal FFT. Accuracy can be improved by exploiting MIMO. Moreover, as discussed in [12], MIMO turns out to be extremely effective for the simultaneous monitoring of the HR of two subjects, thanks to the possibility of identifying the angular dimension of the subject.

A description of the MIMO technology applied to radar systems is contained in [6]. Differently from classic communication systems application, the main goal in a radar context is to increase the angular resolution without adding complexity to the system. As stated in [11], the result is a virtual receiving antenna, whose characteristics depend on the position of the transmitter and the receivers.

4.1 Radar Signal Processing

As described in [3], the HR extraction procedure from radar works as follows. The radar transmits a sequence of chirps divided into frames. Each chirp is designed to be able to precisely detect the position of a subject. It is possible to use only one frame for each chirp, thus not creating a data overhead during the processing phase. It is important to carefully set the duration of each chirp and the number of the contained frames within it, since these values directly impact on the sample rate of the HR. From [10] the sampling frequency along the slow time can be written as

$$f_{sampling[HR]} = \frac{k}{t_{periodicity}}, \tag{4}$$

where k is the number of chirps inside one frame and $t_{periodicity}$ represents the frame duration.

For a better target position identification the MIMO technology is applied. Using this technique is possible to identify not only the distance but also the angle position, this is an improvement of the algorithm accuracy [5,31].

A Field Programmable Gate Array (FPGA) is used to collect the samples of the beat signals from the ADCs. These signals come from four receivers' lines, and it is possible to store the samples in a data cube. This cube is depicted in Fig. 9. Samples of a single chirps are stored along the fast time, samples of different chirps are stored along the slow time, while samples of different receivers are stored along the spatial sampling. The fast time is used to detect the range distance of the subject, the spatial sampling and the slow time detect the angle and the velocity, respectively.

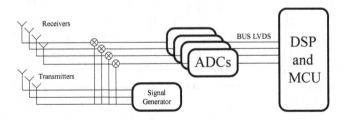

Fig. 8. AWR1843 scheme.

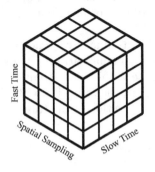

Fig. 9. MIMO data cube [24].

By performing a bi-dimensional FFT on the Fast Time - Spatial Sampling plane, we obtain information about the subject position for each transmitted chirp. In our tests the target is static and there is no great variation in the FFT of the different chirps. In Fig. 10 we show an example of this FFT, where the red square represents the subject.

Once evaluated the target position, it is possible to apply the algorithm for the extraction of the HR. The displacement variation due to the heart contraction is far below the radar range resolution, thus making the phase analysis the only way of extracting the HR. The HR in fact produces a phase modulation of the FFT signal corresponding to the target position, as described in [5]. After this identification is possible to extract the signal of interest along the slow time. The information is inside the phase, for this reason a phase extraction and unwrap operation are needed. After having obtained the phase signal we can filter it in the range of the heartbeat, i.e. between 60 beats/min and 150 beats/min. The values used in our setting are reported in Table 1.

By applying a FFT to the filtered signal it is possible to extract the value of the HR. The highest peak represents the value of the HR. However, a drawback of this method is that in some measurements there are many peaks with similar amplitude, thus making difficult the detection of the correct value. In order to avoid this problem and to improve the detection capability it is possible to apply the MUSIC algorithm [29]. The use of MUSIC results in a pseudo-spectrum. This gives a spectral information of the signal which depends on the size of the vector base chosen. By increasing the size of the base we have again the spectral representation given by the FFT. In the analyzes made by exploiting the FFT it is very rare that the highest peak is that related to the HR. The reason is that the band pass filter used generates very high harmonic components near the lower cut-off frequency. By applying the MUSIC algorithm it is possible to mitigate this effect, so that the highest peak actually represents the correct value of the HR.

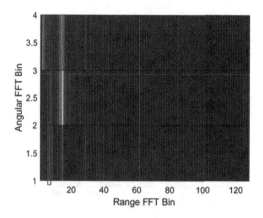

Fig. 10. Subject position identification [24].

Table 1. Filters parameters [24].

Parameter	Value
Filter type	FIR equiripple
f_{stop1}	0.8 Hz
f_{pass1}	1.1 Hz
f_{stop2}	2.5 Hz
f_{pass2}	2.8 Hz

5   Experimental Results

Experimental tests were conducted at the ICT Laboratory of the Polytechnic University of Marche on a set of 16 Caucasian and Asian people of different age and weight. The video is captured with GoPro Hero 6 with a frame rate of 60 fps (2400 frames for a sequence of 40 s) and resolution 1920 × 1080 pixels. Radar and camera were placed on two tripods, radar at a distance of about 20 cm from the subject's chest and GoPro at about 50 cm from the subject's face. The subjects under test were in a standing position. During the video acquisition, the subjects were asked minimize their movements in order to avoid noisy signals or face tracking errors. Videos are captured in indoor conditions, hence we used a standard lamp in addition to the ceiling light to better illuminate the subjects' faces. The physical characteristics of the examined subjects are reported in Table 2.

In Fig. 11 a comparison between the two radar techniques discussed in Sect. 4 is depicted. We observe that the two detection algorithms lead to different results. In the case of the FFT the highest peak corresponds to 64.8 bpm, while in the

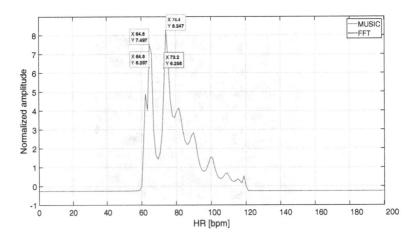

Fig. 11. Extraction comparison between MUSIC and FFT.

Table 2. Physical characteristics of the subjects under test.

Subject [n°]	Characteristics
1	Caucasian
2	Caucasian, Beard
3	Caucasian, Make-up
4	Caucasian, Beard
5	Caucasian
6	Caucasian
7	Caucasian, Tanned
8	Caucasian, Beard
9	Asian
10	Caucasian
11	Caucasian
12	Caucasian, Beard
13	Caucasian
14	Caucasian
15	Caucasian, Make-up
16	Caucasian

case of the MUSIC to 74.4 bpm, which represents the correct value. We note that within the FTT spectrum there is a value around 74 bpm. However, this is not the highest peak, and this affects the detection of the correct HR value.

In Table 3 we report the results achieved by the methodologies described in the previous sections. As regards the radar techniques, in our comparison we do not consider the subjects 13 and 14, since the error is too large. This is probably due to the incorrect position of the radar in front of the subject, which makes difficult to detect the correct target position inside the Angle - Range map. For the cases of the subjects 5, 8 and 15 the value of HR is extracted from the second peak. This problem is also present in the FFT based technique and is a consequence of the filtering process. The application of the MUSIC algorithm makes possible to reduce this effect, so this algorithm improves the performance of the system also from this point of view.

It is possible to evaluate the difference Δ between the two techniques considered and the value measured by the pulse oximeter, averaged over the 16 subjects, using the following equation

$$\Delta_{mean} = \frac{\sum_{n=1}^{N}(POx_n - V_n)}{N}, \tag{5}$$

where N is the number of the subjects, POx represents the value detected by the pulse oximeter and V is the value detected by the applied radar technique.

The MUSIC algorithm results in a Δ_{MUSIC} of -0.227 [bpm], while the FFT in a Δ_{FFT} of 0.157 [bpm]. The two techniques give similar results, but the MUSIC algorithm allows a easier detection of the peak.

In Table 3 we report the characteristics of the subjects (indicated by S) who participated in the tests and the results of the average heartbeat (in bpm) obtained with the considered radar and video methods, with respect to values given by Pulse Oximeter (POx).

Table 3. Tests results on subjects with different physical characteristics. All results are measured in bpm.

S	POx	EVM	ICA(G)	ICA(G)+PCA	ICA+PCA+SD	FFT	MUSIC
1	76	77	72	70	70	77	75.6
2	102	98	98	81	85	98.4	100.8
3	93	98	85	90	91	93.6	91
4	67	64	54	70	57	70	72
5	64	62	70	70	67	64	64.8
6	73	72	72	67	72	73	72
7	93	90	88	76	83	92.4	91.2
8	72	77	67	70	70	71	72
9	73	75	75	90	67	72	70.8
10	81	69	75	90	72	83	81.6
11	78	77	78	79	75	79	80.4
12	103	111	83	104	91	104	103.2
13	72	72	72	70	80	67	/
14	93	95	85	93	93	82	/
15	83	80	80	96	85	80	81.6
16	71	69	70	93	67	73.2	72

In Table 4 we evaluate the mean relative error (MRE) between different methods, taking as a reference value the one measured by the pulse oximeter. As regards the methods based on video processing, we observe that the EVM method is the most accurate but computationally heavy and requires a manual setting of the ROIs. The method which includes the skin detection can instead represent a good trade-off between computational speed, automatism for the real time detection and accuracy. We also note that implementing the MUSIC algorithm allows to reduce the MRE with respect to the use of the FFT.

Table 4. Comparison and percentage error between different methods.

Methods	MRE [%]
POx-EVM	0.55
POx-ICA	6.92
POx-(ICA+PCA)	10.06
POx-(ICA+PCA+SD)	7.71
POx-FFT	2.82
POx-MUSIC	1.86

6   Conclusions

We have compared different contactless methodologies for the heart rate estimation, based on video and radar signal processing of data collected using low cost devices, such as a commercial camera and an automotive radar. Algorithms based on Independent Components Analysis (ICA), Principal Components Analysis (PCA) and Skin Detection have been proposed to improve the computational speed of video processing based on Eulerian Video Magnification (EVM) and to automatize the process, while the MUSIC algorithm has been considered to improve the accuracy in the detection of the heart rate through radar. In particular, the use of ICA, PCA and Skin Detection avoids the manual selection of the ROIs from which to extract the heart rate, thus allowing to realize a real time oriented system, at the expenses of a greater error (but still less than 10%). This represents a good trade-off between precision and efficiency and above all it allows an accurate home monitoring of subjects affected by different pathologies. We have compared the performances achieved by the proposed algorithms with those obtained by a pulse oximeter, taken as a reference, showing the feasibility and the accuracy of the analyzed contactless methodologies.

References

1. Alghoul, K., Alharthi, S., Al Osman, H., El Saddik, A.: Heart rate variability extraction from videos signals: ICA vs. EVM comparison. IEEE Access 5, 4711–4719 (2017)
2. Bolanos, M., Nazeran, H., Haltiwanger, E.: Comparison of heart rate variability signal features derived from electrocardiography and photoplethysmography in healthy individuals. In: 2006 International Conference of the IEEE Engineering in Medicine and Biology Society, pp. 4289–4294 (2006)
3. Ciattaglia, G., Senigagliesi, L., De Santis, A., Ricciuti, M.: Contactless measurement of physiological parameters. In: 2019 IEEE 9th International Conference on Consumer Electronics (ICCE-Berlin), pp. 22–26, September 2019. https://doi.org/10.1109/ICCE-Berlin47944.2019.8966140
4. De Ponte Müller, F.: Survey on ranging sensors and cooperative techniques for relative positioning of vehicles. Sensor 17, 271 (2017)

5. Ding, L., Ali, M., Patole, S., Dabak, A.: Vibration parameter estimation using FMCW radar. In: 2016 IEEE International Conference on Acoustics, Speech and Signal Processing (ICASSP), pp. 2224–2228, March 2016. https://doi.org/10.1109/ICASSP.2016.7472072
6. Fishler, E., Haimovich, A., Blum, R., Chizhik, D., Cimini, L., Valenzuela, R.: MIMO radar: an idea whose time has come. In: Proceedings of the 2004 IEEE Radar Conference (IEEE Cat. No.04CH37509), pp. 71–78, April 2004. https://doi.org/10.1109/NRC.2004.1316398
7. Fletcher, R.R., Chamberlain, D., Paggi, N., Deng, X.: Implementation of smart phone video plethysmography and dependence on lighting parameters. In: 2015 37th Annual International Conference of the IEEE Engineering in Medicine and Biology Society (EMBC), pp. 3747–3750 (2015)
8. Fouad, R.M., Omer, O.A., Aly, M.H.: Optimizing remote photoplethysmography using adaptive skin segmentation for real-time heart rate monitoring. IEEE Access 7, 76513–76528 (2019)
9. Gambi, E., et al.: Heart rate detection using Microsoft Kinect: validation and comparison to wearable devices. Sensors 17(8), 1776 (2017)
10. Instruments, T.: AWR 1843 single-chip 76-GHz to 81-GHz automotive radar sensor evaluation module (2019). http://www.ti.com/tool/AWR1843BOOST
11. Jian, L., Stoica, P.: MIMO Radar Signal Processing, 1st edn. Wiley-IEEE Press (2009)
12. Lee, H., Kim, B.H., Park, J.K., Yook, J.G.: A novel vital-sign sensing algorithm for multiple subjects based on 24-GHz FMCW doppler radar. Remote Sens. 11, 1237 (2019)
13. Lewandowska, M., Rumiński, J., Kocejko, T., Nowak, J.: Measuring pulse rate with a webcam – a non-contact method for evaluating cardiac activity. In: 2011 Federated Conference on Computer Science and Information Systems (FedCSIS), pp. 405–410 (2011)
14. Li, X., Chen, J., Zhao, G., Pietikäinen, M.: Remote heart rate measurement from face videos under realistic situations. In: 2014 IEEE Conference on Computer Vision and Pattern Recognition, pp. 4264–4271, June 2014. https://doi.org/10.1109/CVPR.2014.543
15. Lin, J.C., Kiernicki, J., Kiernicki, M., Wollschlaeger, P.B.: Microwave apexcardiography. IEEE Trans. Microw. Theory Tech. 27(6), 618–620 (1979). https://doi.org/10.1109/TMTT.1979.1129682
16. Madhav, K.V., Ram, M.R., Krishna, E.H., Reddy, K.N., Reddy, K.A.: Estimation of respiratory rate from principal components of photoplethysmographic signals. In: 2010 IEEE EMBS Conference on Biomedical Engineering and Sciences (IECBES), pp. 311–314 (2010)
17. Motin, M.A., Karmakar, C.K., Palaniswami, M.: Ensemble empirical mode decomposition with principal component analysis: a novel approach for extracting respiratory rate and heart rate from photoplethysmographic signal. IEEE J. Biomed. Health Inform. 22(3), 766–774 (2018)
18. Muñoz-Ferreras, J., Wang, J., Peng, Z., Li, C., Gómez-García, R.: FMCW-radar-based vital-sign monitoring of multiple patients. In: 2019 IEEE MTT-S International Microwave Biomedical Conference (IMBioC), vol. 1, pp. 1–3, May 2019. https://doi.org/10.1109/IMBIOC.2019.8777845
19. Peng, R.C., Zhou, X.L., Lin, W.H., Zhang, Y.T.: Extraction of heart rate variability from smartphone photoplethysmograms. Comput. Math. Methods Med. 2015 (2015)

20. Pisa, S., Pittella, E., Piuzzi, E.: A survey of radar systems for medical applications. IEEE Aerosp. Electron. Syst. Mag. **31**(11), 64–81 (2016)
21. Poh, M., McDuff, D.J., Picard, R.W.: Advancements in noncontact, multiparameter physiological measurements using a webcam. IEEE Trans. Biomed. Eng. **58**(1), 7–11 (2011)
22. Ram, M.R., Madhav, K.V., Krishna, E.H., Reddy, K.N., Reddy, K.A.: Use of multiscale principal component analysis for motion artifact reduction of PPG signals. In: 2011 IEEE Recent Advances in Intelligent Computational Systems, pp. 425–430 (2011)
23. Ren, L., Wang, H., Naishadham, K., Kilic, O., Fathy, A.E.: Phase-based methods for heart rate detection using UWB impulse doppler radar. IEEE Trans. Microw. Theory Tech. **64**(10), 3319–3331 (2016). https://doi.org/10.1109/TMTT. 2016.2597824
24. Ricciuti, M., Ciattaglia, G., De Santis, A., Gambi, E., Senigagliesi, L.: Contactless heart rate measurements using RGB-camera and radar. In: ICT4AWE, pp. 121–129 (2020)
25. Rumiński, J.: Reliability of pulse measurements in videoplethysmography. Metrol. Measur. Syst. **23**(3) (2016)
26. Secerbegovic, A., Bergsland, J., Halvorsen, P.S., Suljanovic, N., Mujcic, A., Balasingham, I.: Blood pressure estimation using video plethysmography. In: 2016 IEEE 13th International Symposium on Biomedical Imaging (ISBI), pp. 461–464 (2016)
27. Wang, S., Pohl, A., Jaeschke, T., Czaplik, M., Köny, M., Leonhardt, S., Pohl, N.: A novel ultra-wideband 80 GHz FMCW radar system for contactless monitoring of vital signs. In: 2015 37th Annual International Conference of the IEEE Engineering in Medicine and Biology Society (EMBC), pp. 4978–4981, August 2015. https://doi.org/10.1109/EMBC.2015.7319509
28. Wang, Y., Liu, Q., Fathy, A.E.: CW and pulse-doppler radar processing based on FPGA for human sensing applications. IEEE Trans. Geosci. Remote Sens. **51**(5), 3097–3107 (2013). https://doi.org/10.1109/TGRS.2012.2217975
29. Wang, Y., Wang, W., Zhou, M., Ren, A., Tian, Z.: Remote monitoring of human vital signs based on 77-GHz mm-wave FMCW radar. Sensors **20**(10), 2999 (2020)
30. Wu, H.Y., Rubinstein, M., Shih, E., Guttag, J., Durand, F., Freeman, W.: Eulerian video magnification for revealing subtle changes in the world. ACM Trans. Graph. **31**(4), 1–8 (2012)
31. Xiong, Y., Peng, Z., Xing, G., Zhang, W., Meng, G.: Accurate and robust displacement measurement for FMCW radar vibration monitoring. IEEE Sens. J. **18**(3), 1131–1139 (2018). https://doi.org/10.1109/JSEN.2017.2778294

Ontology-Driven Mental Healthcare Applications: A Case Study on Cognitive Rehabilitation with Serious Games

Christos Goumopoulos[✉] and Ioannis Igoumenakis

Information and Communication Systems Engineering Department, University of the Aegean, Samos, Greece
goumop@aegean.gr, i.igoumenakis@gmail.com

Abstract. The emergence of Semantic Web offered an opportunity for developing new approaches regarding the integration, deployment and operation of healthcare applications. By combining network connectivity, contemporary software architectural styles and semantic-based technologies efficient representation and communication of data and knowledge is feasible between different system components. In this context, standards such as Resource Description Framework (RDF) and Web Ontology Language (OWL) are underpinning the definition of ontologies in the healthcare domain. The aim of this work is to provide insights on the design and implementation of ontology-based healthcare applications. The focus is on the domain of mental healthcare and in particular the development of a game platform for mild cognitive impairment rehabilitation is examined closely as a case study. The positive impact of the synergy between healthcare applications and ontologies is discussed and some of the major challenges and obstacles in this scope are identified.

Keyword: Ontology · Semantic web · Serious games · Mental health · Microservices

1 Introduction

A difficult problem regarding the realization of healthcare applications is the provision of interoperability between the different system components involved [1]. The importance of this requirement is associated with the need to realize a universal understanding of the involved knowledge, to support the integration of heterogeneous information, to provide responses to complex questions, as well as to cater for data integration and knowledge exchange in the healthcare context. Due to such requirements, and also in order to enable the distribution of health-related information between different administration entities, the Semantic Web can support the possibility of exchanging such information among different healthcare systems. This is accomplished by using ontologies to create a common language for efficient information representation, as well as Web standards to enable interoperability in the transmission of information [2].

© Springer Nature Switzerland AG 2021
M. Ziefle et al. (Eds.): ICT4AWE 2020, CCIS 1387, pp. 114–140, 2021.
https://doi.org/10.1007/978-3-030-70807-8_7

Ontology, in the context of the Semantic Web, is defined as the vocabulary, terminology and relationships between concepts of a thematic area [3]. The ontology provides the meaning and context to the information available on the Internet resources for an application domain and consists of two parts: i) the *Schema*, i.e. the concepts that obey an hierarchy between them, as well as the associations (roles) between them; and ii) the *Data*, which are the instances of these structural elements. At the same time, each ontology should be described with explicit formal semantics using a logical language and should be characterized by logical coherence, as well as by semantic coverage, in order to be able to cover all entities in the specified field [4]. In addition, it should offer modeling accuracy by enabling representation only of models intended for the field of interest, strong modularity by providing an organization of its theories for the conceptual field, and finally, scalability, by adopting a language that allows to express efficiently all the proposed concepts.

Consequently, the ontology of each field should contain an organization of classes, objects, and their relationships, along with inferential rules. This common understanding of concepts and relationships allows the integration of knowledge between different healthcare systems. However, although ontologies denote the conceptual foundation for the modeling of information, consistent data transmission between different systems is achieved with the help of standards. The data, which are contained within closed healthcare systems come in various forms. The necessary healthcare knowledge, however, must be accessible. This can be achieved through the adoption of appropriate interoperability standards which can empower information integration enabling transparency in healthcare-related processes, including all necessary system entities.

The most basic standard of Semantic Web interoperability is the Resource Description Framework (RDF) [5], which is an object-aware template that provides reusable data for data exchange through the Internet. Its uniqueness lies in the fact that each concept has a Uniform Resource Identifier (URI), which in turn identifies each element of the Web, thus avoiding any semantic ambiguity. Furthermore, in order to express the representations of an ontology for a specific domain, RDF permits construct additions leading to other formulations such as the OWL (Web Ontology Language) standard [6].

An ontology, can be formally described in OWL using classes, objects, and properties as key attributes. These elements are used to describe concepts, instances or members of a class, as well as relationships between objects of two different classes (*object properties*), and can also be used to associate objects with data types (*data type properties*). In addition to these key elements, however, the OWL language also provides descriptions of each class used to accurately describe OWL classes, which in turn include data on property constraints, class axioms, and properties that concern each person individually.

On the other hand, the existence of rules contributes to the combination of the knowledge of an ontology with corresponding dynamic knowledge, which are included in these rules [7]. A system based on the use of rules usually contains a set of "if-then" rules that indicate the next action to be made, depending on the situation, but also a rule mechanism used to enforce them. Thus, the use of a set of rules makes it possible to express the behavior of individuals within a field, thus providing new knowledge about these individuals and, consequently, personalized services [8].

Therefore, an ontology can be a semantic repository for the management of the knowledge model that includes information related to the application domain, related to the environment in which the application is available. In this way, for example, it is possible for disease management applications to analyze the data related to the symptoms and the relevant profile of the patient (medical history, age, etc.) and thus, to suggest the necessary interventions each time (e.g., a program of using games/memory exercises in patients with memory loss).

This study presents an overview of representative ontology-based healthcare systems with a special focus on a case study on cognitive rehabilitation using serious games. More specifically, the next section provides insights on the design and implementation of existing ontology-based healthcare applications focusing on mental healthcare. Then, an ontology-based game platform for mild cognitive impairment rehabilitation is presented in more detail. The positive impact of the synergy between healthcare applications and ontologies is discussed and some of the major challenges and obstacles in this scope are identified. Finally, this work concludes with a comprehensive evaluation of using ontologies as a method of improving healthcare, as well as future challenges that may arise along the way.

2 Ontology Driven Healthcare Applications

2.1 Remote Health Monitoring

The first healthcare application examined concerns an ontology-based health monitoring system for home-based scenarios that allows to integrate and manage relevant data [9]. The ontology-based remote health monitoring system architecture is divided into two layers. The first layer is the conceptual layer and the second is the data and communication layer. The conceptual layer deals with the representation of data while the second layer deals with data management and transmission. From a deployment perspective, the remote monitoring system includes a Telemonitoring Server located on the health-care side, and several Home Gateways located on the home sites. Communication between the two end points (Gateways and Server) is achieved through a Web Service, installed in the Server and a Web Client, installed in the Gateway. This architecture enables communication through the HTTPS protocol and is used to provide monitoring services for patients with chronic diseases, as well as to support remote management of Medical Devices.

At the conceptual layer, the two endpoints of the remote monitoring scenario must address heterogeneous data gathered from different devices. The aim of the developed ontology was to model both the data involved and their management process. Therefore, the produced ontology denotes the common knowledge required to realize the integration of the two end points of the architecture as well as to support their communication mechanism. A general ontology, called HOTMES (Home ontology for integrated management in home-based scenarios), was first designed to describe the general management of the remote monitoring system, and then two ontology extensions were delivered, the HOTMES clinical and the HOTMES technical (Fig. 1).

The primary goal of using the HOTMES ontology is to provide a general framework to define a management profile which includes four different tasks: a) monitoring, b) analysis, c) planning, and d) execution. Using this idea, Home Gateway provides to some extent the possibility of autonomous behavior. Depending on the content of the management profile, a Gateway will be able to monitor the information provided by various sources, analyze the information obtained (in relation to the rules used in the analysis task), to react to non-physiological states and report changes in environmental information. In this context, a set of rules are given along with the management profile to specify when the analysis output provides an alarm or not and when the planning function should be activated (e.g. to schedule actions to address adverse events).

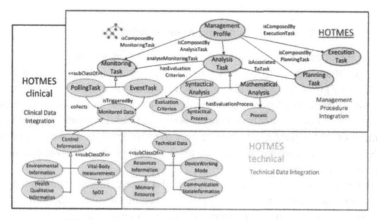

Fig. 1. HOTMES ontology and its main classes [9].

At the data level, communication between endpoints is done using Web Services (WS) technologies. REST WS was developed to improve the scalability and flexibility of the system architecture and to improve its performance. The WS includes and defines a set of actions on the following resources: an OWL ontology, rules (transmitted via XML), OWL objects, datatype value properties corresponding to an object and informational messages, to support certain control functions in communication between endpoints. Each of these resources is recognized by a URI, and also has a set of functions via HTTP methods such as GET and PUT). Jena framework was used to edit the ontology and create new instances, obtain data, and manipulate the application of the rules.

To evaluate the effectiveness of the proposed system, two management profiles on clinical and technical management tasks were designed for a patient with Chronic Obstructive Pulmonary Disease (COPD). Therefore, a patient profile was designed according to the HOTMES clinical ontology and a technical management profile was designed according to the HOTMES technical ontology. The patient profile includes the tasks required to monitor a COPD patient, such as the device measurement to detect the presence and severity of airway obstruction. The patient profile was developed by a primary care physician following published clinical guidelines and included 15 monitoring tasks, 11 analysis tasks, 9 planning tasks and 3 execution tasks. This configuration led to the creation of 144 new class instances and the configuration of 18 rules [10].

To evaluate the system architecture two tests were performed. First, the COPD profiles in the case study were used, and connections and data transfers between the client and the WS were simulated in order to obtain the profiles and related rules. In this test the performance of the architecture was evaluated in terms of network cost and execution time. The second test concerned the execution in combination of both the COPD patient profile and the technical management profile. The system was evaluated in terms of computational and memory cost. To activate the alarms defined in the management profile, and thus to demonstrate the functionality of the system, the data from the Medical Devices and the Gateway were simulated. After the initial setup, all simulated alarm events were detected by the system and therefore the relevant actions were successfully performed.

2.2   Interventions to Address Dementia Related Behaviors

The second healthcare application explored is founded on human-centered models of dementia care that emphasize the importance of addressing individual needs and emotional responses [11]. The approach examined focuses on an intervention system that uses pervasive computing technologies to improve patients' quality of life by detecting the presence of dementia, deciding on appropriate intervention by either modifying the environment or persuading the patient or caregiver to act in accordance with system advice. System services are tailored to the specific needs of the caregiver and the person suffering from the disease.

The development of the ontologies followed a user-centered methodology which allowed knowledge engineers to understand the specific field with the participation of users and experts in this domain. The approach includes an initial stage of understanding, which consists of reviewing the relevant literature on the field from which the concepts and relationships of the ontology are derived. Use case scenarios were derived from interviews and observations from relevant studies. These scenarios demonstrated the diversity of problematic behaviors associated with the disease and the need for personal intervention by assisting the patients and their caregiver.

The developed ontology is organized in multiple layers as illustrated in Fig. 2. The upper-layer is a domain ontology that provides a general understanding of the types of dementia a patient may experience (e.g., wandering, agitation and apathy), the type of factors that have a direct effect on these behaviors, or which event triggers them. These factors are determined by the caregiver by observing their manifestations and by adopting an appropriate intervention. The lower ontology layer extends some concepts of the upper layer, which are used to decide which intervention will be recommended or implemented. A multi-layered ontology facilitates its expansion by adding specialized knowledge about: a) the particular factors that may produce dementia behaviors or influence intervention choice, e.g., personality and the patient's demographic profile; the period before the disease; b) the different treatments that can be applied to the intervention, e.g. a sensory intervention may include listening to music; c) the particular features of dementia, e.g., wandering patterns suggesting measurable properties; and d) the observed manifestations of a dementia behavior, such as verbal assault or repetitive peculiarities.

System services are used to help caregivers and patients deal with problematic behaviors, and to suggest appropriate interventions for the caregiver or to apply them directly to the environment. Decisions to treat dementia and the intervention to be used are supported by the developed ontology. The ontology supports the adaptation of services in two stages. On the one hand, during knowledge engineering the ontology offers the opportunity to tailor system services to a patient and caregiver. On the other hand, during development, the context information collected by the sensors in the environment or explicitly recorded by the caregiver or patient is used to trigger opportunistic interventions.

The ontology includes also the definition of decision rules to determine the intervention that must be provided by the system and the rules that will allow the system to decide on the type of intervention it will propose or activate. The system can assess the presence of dementia behavior through opportunistic detection or respond to an explicit dementia report from the caregiver. When an incidence of dementia occurs, the system refers to the ontology to match between an intervention and the current case. For example, there are rules for adapting the patient's atmosphere and rules for personalizing the intervention according to the patient's current context and parameters so that if the patient is in another patient's room, then the system should perform the intervention by notifying the caregiver.

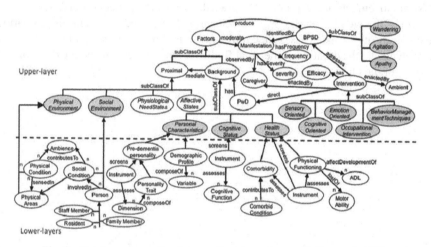

Fig. 2. Ontology supporting interventions to patients with Dementia [11].

The evaluation of the ontology-based system was performed with a two month intervention with a patient and a caregiver to assess the effectiveness and usefulness of the approach. The main dementia behaviors concerning the evaluation were disorientation, apathy and lack of independence to comply with a medication protocol. The caregiver was asked to keep a written diary based on cards reporting incidents of problematic behaviors. To customize system services, an ontology instance was created with the information collected by the caregiver.

2.3 Home Care for Patients with Alzheimer

As the interest to integrate new technologies such as pervasive computing and sensor networks in healthcare grows, one area of focus is the development of systems targeting behavioral understanding based on activities-of-daily-living (ADL) of patients. Such systems can facilitate home care and clinical evaluation of elderly patients with Alzheimer. The application discussed in this section describes an approach to achieve such a goal by providing a reusable middleware based on Semantic Web standards [12].

The behavioral understanding targeted by the particular system was related to the automated quantification of patient confusion. The wide range of contexts associated with this quantification is categorized into three sub-ontologies: (a) assessment/observation of confusion in people with Alzheimer, (b) intervention and (c) social semantics. More specifically, the confusion assessment/observation model was used to classify the degree of confusion experienced by a person with Alzheimer. This tool consists of seven scaled elements (i.e., body/up and down movements, repetitive/outward motions, loud words, repetitive vocalization and negative words) each object representing an observable behavior. At intervals of five minutes, the duration of the patient's physical movements and expressions is graded. The overall patient observation score is the sum of the weights of all observed behaviors. More specifically, in Fig. 3a part of the ontology of confusion assessment/observation is shown consisting of two representative elements: the duration of the Total Body Movement element and the duration and intensity of the Outward motion.

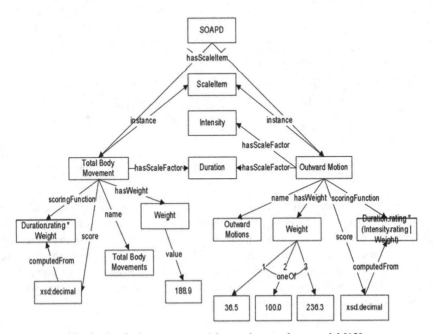

Fig. 3. Confusion assessment/observation ontology model [12].

Since the system can automatically distinguish a patient who is upset, predictions can be made to achieve timely therapeutic interventions, defining the corresponding ontology of interventions. For example, relaxing music was thought to help an upset patient to calm down. Therefore, if a patient is identified with a mild degree of confusion, then the system automatically activates music therapy to calm him or her down, as initially defined by the caregiver.

The social context ontology is defined for those cases where the patient does not respond to treatment such as the relaxing music and is increasingly upset; therefore, the system must inform the patient's caregiver of this condition. At the same time, in case the person caring for the patient is not available at the given time, due to an important obligation, the system informs the next caregiver, using the FOAF (Friend Of A Friend) ontology [13].

The ontology knowledge base includes a repository using SeQRL (Sesame RDF Query Language) as the query language. A query mechanism provides an abstract interface to the applications so that all the desired frames can be extracted. The inference mechanism consists of a wide range of techniques, which can range from rule systems to neural networks and fuzzy logic, to improve the decision-making process by injecting appropriate rules or logic. Social resources include email, calendar, and social media applications, which can be combined to find new indirect social media links.

3   Cognitive Rehabilitation

3.1   Serious Games

Serious Games (SG) have been used intensively in the field of healthcare for treatment and rehabilitation purposes [14]. In recent years, due to the increasing rate of people suffering from cognitive impairment, such as the elderly adults with Mild Cognitive Impairment (MCI) [15], SG have been the focus of research targeting physical as well as mental exercising in order to reduce and gradually eliminate the symptoms of such conditions [16]. In this context, the main purpose of SG is to help the elderly to remain mentally, physically and socially active by providing to them the appropriate stimuli.

The recovery of cognitive impairments is traditionally performed with written exercises (pen and paper method), in which the patient is asked to answer in writing or orally a series of questions. This method requires a lot of effort on the side of the professionals who supervise the rehabilitation process and need to constantly adjust the difficulty of the exercises to the level of the patient by creating different exercises that ultimately keep the patient interested to the process. Furthermore there is a need to cater for the collection and storage of statistical data generated by the process and which could be used to study the performance and evolution of methods. The idea behind the use of SG in cognitive rehabilitation is that the automatically generated exercises will be more attractive to the patients and so they will interact with them with greater dedication and more frequently.

Therefore, the use of SG could become low-cost interventions that can provide significant assistance in delaying or even stopping the cognitive impairment in older people. In order to achieve an effective result, it is necessary to frame the proper design of the games by involving a multidisciplinary team, for example, taking into account neurophysiological scientific knowledge and learning theories, but also considering the feedback that will result from the interested end users. However, the scope of SG related to cognitive rehabilitation has not been fully mapped, so it is necessary to further research and evaluate more such games, especially those designed primarily for the entertainment of ordinary people but which in the process proved to be positive in terms of the treatment of MCI.

In that respect, recent studies have focused on the use of SG for cognitive rehabilitation in order for the recovery to be done faster and more successfully, without at the same time tiring the patient psychologically [17]. Mobile computing technologies are used to automate the written exercises used until recently, by providing the patient with a variety of different stimuli such as words, sounds and images. Furthermore, the rehabilitation specialists are supported in that way by providing to them greater ease in planning and evaluating the course of treatment.

3.2   COGNIPLAT Platform

The COGNIPLAT platform (https://cogniplat.aegean.gr/) is an innovative cognitive impairment rehabilitation tool that is developed for assisting elderly who have MCI but have not yet developed dementia. It is built based on a multi-disciplinary approach combining theories of neuropsychology, cognitive linguistics and speech therapy focused on enhancing cognitive functions through different game exercises. In addition, the platform has been designed to adjust the complexity and type of exercises by adapting the cognitive requirements of the games to the characteristics of each patient.

The large number of stimuli of the COGNIPLAT platform (text, image, sound) allows great variation in the exercises, something that would be impossible with the method of written exercises used in the past. It is practically impossible for a patient to see an exercise repeated a second time with the same stimuli (same words to recognize). This helps maintain the patient's interest and motivation to continue the process for a long time.

The term cognitive skills refers to the actions that the human brain needs to take in order for a person to be able to think and learn. Such skills include memory function (short and long term), the ability to process visual/auditory stimuli and reasoning (to be able to draw logical conclusions depending on the situations). The concept of cognitive rehabilitation does not imply curing the cause of the dysfunction. The main goal of the methodology is to train the patient's cognitive function so that it can respond in the desired way to the stimuli.

Currently fifteen games have been implemented as shown in Table 1 where the targeted cognitive area is also indicated. All games effectively practice skills that include hand-eye coordination, memory, language, following instructions, comprehension, object recognition, sustained attention and praxis (i.e., the ability to perform skillful movements indicating the operation of primary sensory and motor organs).

Table 1. COGNILAT platform games.

Game	Description	Cognitive area
Anagram	Solving a word puzzle	Reasoning
Antonyms & Synonyms	Finding word antonyms/synonyms	Memory
Calculation	Solving arithmetic crosswords	Reasoning
ChronologicalOrder	Placing shuffled images in chronological order in order to create a brief story	Reasoning
FindThePattern	Remembering a pattern of highlighted boxes appeared shortly in the context of a background screen of boxes	Visual memory
FindTheSound	Listening to sounds and selecting the corresponding image	Acoustic memory
Labyrinth	Finding the exit from a labyrinth	Perception
LogicalOrder	Selecting the right pattern to reasonably complete the given sequence	Reasoning
MemoryCards	Revealing pairs of alike pictures	Memory
NumberOrder	Ordering a random sequence of numbers in increasing sequence	Reasoning
Observation	Counting specific types of objects given a set of discrete images shown on the screen	Attention
Outsider	Finding an object that does not match with the rest	Attention
Puzzle	Solving a photo puzzle	Attention
Quiz	Recalling knowledge in various categories such as history, geography, food, etc.	Memory
Suitcase	Placing an object in the correct position so that the suitcase closes without collisions with existing objects	Perception

The patients may use the platform at home either independently or together with a family member or a caregiver in case of severe cognitive impairment. The user interface design has been developed taking into account the characteristics of the elderly which call for simplicity, clarity, consistency and adaptability to the skills of each individual [18]. Figure 4 shows the user interface of two example games.

Figure 5 shows, as another example, the user interface for the *Suitcase* game. In this game, an open suitcase is displayed on a table with some objects placed on both sides. The user is asked to put a new object in the proper place so that the suitcase closes without the objects that are on either side of it are colliding with each other. The size of the suitcase as well as the items change depending on the level of difficulty.

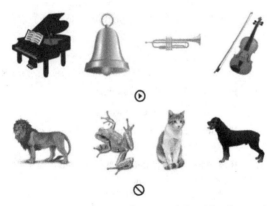

Fig. 4. Snapshots from *FindTheSound* (top) and *Outsider* (bottom) games [17].

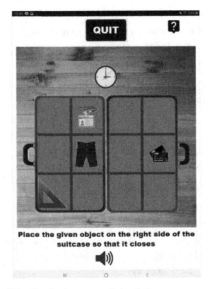

Fig. 5. An instance of the *Suitcase* game.

3.3 Ontologies

Each ontology language has a specific amount of expressiveness. OWL by having many features leads to high expressiveness, which in turn leads to computational cost. To tackle this issue, OWL can adjust its expressiveness levels by using a specific profile. OWL provides three profiles OWL Full, OWL DL and OWL Lite [19], while OWL2 introduced three new OWL 2 EL, OWL 2 QL and OWL 2 RL [20]. In this work, the OWL 2 DL (Description Logic) profile was used to specify the ontology models.

In this context, the SPARQL (SPARQL Protocol and RDF Query Language) language was used to query the knowledge base of the ontology and to describe rules that encode expressions over the user profile instances. Despite being a query language,

SPARQL provides extensive power to guide the provision of personalized services by filtering persons with certain characteristics (applying the FILTER NOT EXISTS construct), asserting new facts (applying the CONSTRUCT expression), updating data in the ontology (applying the UPDATE expression), asking or selecting the existence of an individual or of a complicated relation (applying the ASK or SELECT expression accordingly), etc. Therefore, personalized game activities can be defined via SPARQL rules according to user conditions and preferences.

Protégé (v. 5.5.0) ontology editor was used to create the ontologies. Protégé is a software tool that enables the creation of an OWL ontology and supports the capabilities of the OWL language. Protégé supports the definition of a hierarchy of *entities-classes* as well as the ability to create *relationships-restrictions* via a handy graphical user interface instead of directly using the OWL language. Moreover, it allows the import of remote ontologies and the display of their classes and properties. Extending from there it allows the creation of new relations or classes which can inherit or relate with these imported entities, meaning classes or properties. It also comes integrated with various reasoners, which control the consistency of the ontology as well as infer new knowledge. In this work the Pellet reasoner, an open source Java OWL-DL reasoner, was chosen. Finally, it provides useful ontology information such as the set of axioms, i.e. the self-proven values, which exist in the ontology.

For a selected entity, Protégé lists the relationships with the following syntax which is adopted in the next sections:

<relationship-name> <cardinality> <cardinality value (optional)> <range of relationship>

where *<cardinality>* may be one of the following keywords: *min, max, exactly, only*.

The following notation is also used for expressing relationships: *OP* denotes *Object-Property* relationships, *DP* denotes *DataProperty* relationships and *obj* denotes all entities that are objects. For example, the following restriction: *hasMathOperation (OP) max 5 MathOperator (obj)*, is interpreted as the *hasMathOperation* relationship is an *ObjectProperty* with *max* cardinality the number 5 of the *MathOperator* entity-object.

User Profile. In COGNIPLAT platform, there is a need for describing, in addition to the static user traits, dynamic aspects that relate to specific game activities in which the user engages. The *User Profile (UP)* uses temporary sub-profiles of a user profile in order to encode game activity related user preferences. Figure 6 depicts the relations between *Person, Profile, TemporarySubProfile* and *PermanentSubprofile* and the properties of each sub-profile. In particular, a Person has exactly one permanent sub-profile and several temporary sub-profiles.

Leveraging on UP data the game platform can select favourably game resources that are aligned to the stored preferences of each patient (e.g. favourite sports, food, hobbies, animals, music, etc.). This personalization of the exercises can increase user engagement and platform acceptability. Similarly, the declared educational level can adjust the exercise parameters (e.g. completion time, performance threshold to change the difficulty level) and exercise plans (e.g., minimize the use of certain games) according to the patient capabilities.

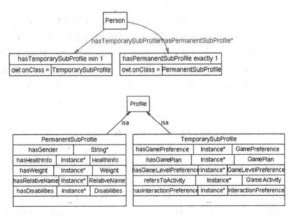

Fig. 6. Visualisation of a part of the UP Ontology [17].

Games. The main goal of the games ontologies is to represent the knowledge of the game rules and their constituent resources so that game instances can be automatically created by an application server. The ontologies also enable the correlation between resources, resulting in a greater variety of entities that can be associated to the rules of the game. The ability to associate entities with one another can lead to new games, such as finding the sound that can characterize a word.

After analyzing the logic of the fifteen MCI rehabilitation games some basic properties have been identified:

- There are different difficulty levels for a game;
- There is a time limit to play a game;
- There is a maximum number of repetitions for a game;
- After a number of correct answers the difficulty level of a game increases;
- A game is associated with resources that can be words, operators, blocks, puzzle pieces, questions, images, videos and sounds.

The games ontologies are structured in a hierarchical way. However, following the bottom up approach may lead to ontology duplication. To resolve this, a base Game ontology introduced that contains a Game class. Also, this ontology introduces the following global datatype properties:

1. *maxCompletionTime (DP) value n*, specifying the time allowed to complete the exercise which can vary depending on the difficulty level of the game. The value is an integer corresponding to a time measured in seconds.
2. *completedDate (DP) value xsd: string*, specifying the end date of the current game.
3. *hasDifficulty (DP) value {"EASY", "MEDIUM", "HARD"}*, specifying the difficulty of the game.
4. *hasGameId (DP) value xsd: string*, specifying a unique identifier of the individual game. The syntax of such an identifier is: *<game name>_<difficulty level>_<player name> _<round number>*.

5. *hasLevel (DP) value xsd: string*, specifying the current level of the game.
6. *hasPlayer (DP) value xsd: string*, specifying the player's alias.
7. *isCompletedIn (DP) value xsd: positiveInteger*, specifying the time in secs for completing the current game.

For each game, a separate ontology is defined. Each game ontology imports the base Game ontology and the requested Resources ontologies based on the resources that it requires. Each game class inherits from the imported Game class the global properties. Moreover, each game class has access to the classes of the resources that have been imported and therefore can define relations-restrictions with them. Finally, each game ontology defines a base class that represents the core rules and subclasses representing a different difficulty level. As an example, the entity in Fig. 7 describes the game of associating images to sounds (*FindTheSound*). The number of images displayed in this game increases with respect to the difficulty level. The restrictions (object properties) defined in the ontology for the *FindTheSound* Game entity are as follows:

1. *hasImage (OP) exactly n ImageSound (obj)*, specifying the number of images to be used as options with the associated sound.
2. *hasSound (OP) exactly 1 Sound (obj)*, specifying the sound the user hears with the associated image.

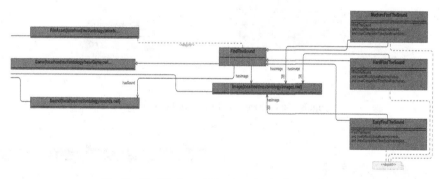

Fig. 7. *FindTheSound* Game entity in the ontology.

For the ontologies of the resources a bottom-up approach is followed. At the bottom there is each resource isolated, with their own data properties, or object properties which their domain and range are the same resource. For example the Word Ontology (Fig. 8) contains classes that are associated directly by the class Word and as well as the object properties *Antonym (D: Word, R: Word)*, *hasSynonym (D: Word, R: Word)* that target an instance of the class word. In the levels above, other ontologies can import any number of resources ontologies and create new object relations between different resources or super classes composed by these individual classes. For example, the ontology FileAssets creates a new superclass named FileAsset of the two imported classes Image and Sound (Fig. 9). Furthermore it defines a class restriction *hasAssetPath(DP)* which is inherited by the imported classes Image and Sound. Moreover, it associates the imported classes with two inverse object properties called *hasAssociatedImage(OP)* and *hasAssociatedSound(OP)*.

This methodology helps with the scalability of the resources as new super classes and relations can be created easily. Another benefit of this approach is that at the bottom levels, the computational complexity is low as the reasoner has fewer classes and properties to infer from and thus less results. On the contrary the top levels have bigger computational complexity but produce more inferred results.

At the top level there is the Resources ontology which defines relationships that associate resources with other resources. A subset of these relationships is provided next in the following format: *relationship (D: Domain, R: Range):*

hasAssociatedSound(D:Image, R:Sound)
hasAssociatedImage(D:Sound, R:Image)
hasBlock(D:BlockSet, R:Block)
hasCategory(D:Question, R:Word)
hasChoice(D:Question, R:Word)

hasConnectingPiece(D:Piece, R:Piece)
hasPiece(D:Puzzle, R:Piece)
hasSubject(D:Image or Sound, R:Word)
hasTitle(D:Image or Sound, R:Word)

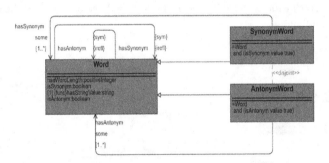

Fig. 8. Visualization of the Word Ontology.

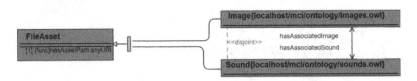

Fig. 9. Visualization of the FileAsset Ontology.

Figure 10 describes, as an example, the Image class, which is required by the game FindTheSound. Each image is associated via the OP relationships *hasTitle* and *hasSubject* with a couple of *Word* entities. In this way, an image can be categorized based on the *hasSubject* relationship and consequently rules can be defined that require images from a specific category. Also, in this manner, games that focus on a *Word* entity can contain rules with corresponding images, such as finding opposite emotions. The *Image* entity is analysed into two subcategories:

1. *OrderedImage*, describing one image and its association with another image via the OP relationship *hasPreviousImage*. It was observed in the developed games that each image may have at most one precursor, which actually characterizes the property as *Functional* (i.e. any entity that belongs to the domain of this relationship can be associated at most with one entity, which belongs to the range of the relationship).
2. *ImageSound*, describing the association of an image with a sound via the OP relationship *hasAssociatedSound*.

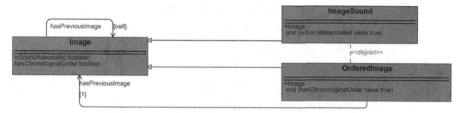

Fig. 10. Image Resource entity in the ontology.

The game ontologies developed currently contains 103 entities with 36 OP relationships and 46 DP relationships. Table 2 shows the reported metrics of the developed ontology. The complete ontology is available in the Github repository (https://github.com/Binarios/MciOntology).

Table 2. Game ontologies metrics.

Category		Value
Metrics	Axiom	746
	Logical axiom	563
	Declaration axiom	183
	Class	103
	Object property	37
	Data property	46
Class axioms	SubClassOf	171
	EquivalentClasses	69
	DisjointClasses	25
	Hidden GCI	55

(continued)

Table 2. (*continued*)

Category		Value
Object property axioms	SubObjectPropertyOf	36
	InverseObjectProperties	1
	DisjointObjectProperties	1
	FunctionalObjectProperty	11
	SymmetricObjectProperty	4
	IrreflexiveObjectProperty	7
	ObjectPropertyDomain	36
	ObjectPropertyRange	36
Data property axioms	SubDataPropertyOf	45
	EquivalentDataProperties	1
	FunctionalDataProperty	30
	DataPropertyDomain	45
	DataPropertyRange	45

3.4 Game Engine

In this section the back end of the COGNIPLAT platform which generates game instances for MCI rehab client applications is described. The COGNIPLAT platform embraces the *microservices architectural style* to deploy game applications as lightweight services that can be independently developed, tested, deployed, operated, scaled, and upgraded [26]. It uses the Kubernetes platform for the deployment of the microservices and *Istio* for controlling incoming and outcoming traffic as well as the traffic between the microservices. The microservices are having the following patterns:

1. *knowledge-base-connector*
2. **-rules*
3. **-nodes*
4. **-provider*

where * is either one of the games or one of the resources. Figure 11 describes the architecture of the platform.

The COGNIPLAT platform uses a cluster-external Apache Jena Fuseki server as the TDB Knowledge-Base in order to achieve persistency of the graph. Also, Fuseki serves the ontologies requested by the **-rules* microservices. This server supports the SPARQL Protocol which makes feasible the communication between the COGNIPLAT platform

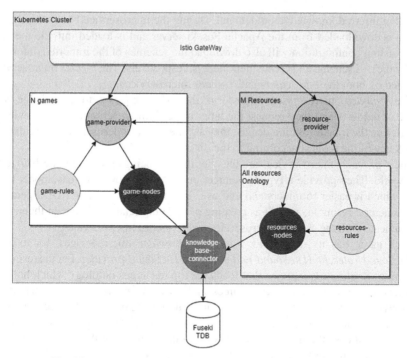

Fig. 11. COGNIPLAT platform microservices-based architecture.

and the Knowledge-Base. Each microservice consists of one embedded Tomcat server for running their functionality. The design pattern that followed for the development is the *dependency injection* (DI). This design pattern increases the decoupling between classes of an application thus achieving greater isolation between them, easier testing of their functionality as well as support for the microservices architecture [27].

The *knowledge-base-connector* microservice hides from the rest of microservices the ontology structure and storage. In this way it is possible to change the ontology technology without disturbing the rest of the system. Moreover, *Istio* can define access rules for each outgoing traffic from the cluster, so the access to the Knowledge Base can be done only by the *knowledge-base-connector* microservice. This microservices is called by the **-nodes* microservices and only during the bootstrap phase by the **-rules* microservices.

The **-rules* microservices are using the Apache Jena API to parse the loaded ontology. The accompanied Apache Jena provides three different APIs. The RDF API supports the creation and reading of RDF triplets. Another API deals with Apache Fuseki functionality as well as the dynamic management of the knowledge base. Finally, the OWL API offers tools and methods to create and access rules in the ontology. The OWL API also provides access to the Pellet reasoner enabling flexibility to the game application by exploiting inferred knowledge on demand. During the microservice bootstrap, the owl schema is downloaded from the Apache Fuseki server and is loaded into the memory. The bootstrap configuration will also download the schemas of the imported ontologies used by the owl schema and create their models, respectively. The *-*rules* microservices are called by both the *-*providers* and *-*nodes* microservices.

The *-*nodes* microservices transform incoming requests to knowledge-base-connector requests and they request the latter to perform an action on the knowledge-base. Before the transformation occurs, they ask the *-*rules* microservice to validate the consistency of the request according to the ontology.

The *-*provider* microservices are the ones that are being exposed by the *Istio* to the outer world. They provide a typed resource, instead of a knowledge-base node, to the caller, which is easier to understand and use. The providers trigger CRUD operations for a game or a resource, as well as creating or updating relations between them. They communicate with the *-*rules* microservices and *-*nodes* microservices.

Each game has its own *rules, nodes* and *provider* microservices, for example *findTheSound-rules, findTheSound-nodes* and *findTheSound-provider*. For the resources, there are one *rules* microservice that loads the top resources ontology which holds all the object properties between the resources, and one *nodes* microservice. Each resource has its own *provider* microservice which can communicate between them to implement the defined restrictions-relations. For example, an Image requires to be associated with a Word. In that case the image-provider will communicate with the words-provider in order to get a word id with which the relation will happen.

The client application (e.g. a health application, an agent, a healthcare expert through a front-end tool) can only access the games services and not the ontology service. Because the services have their own API gateways for communicating with each other, it is necessary to create a master API gateway that only exports the gaming services gateways. The *Istio Gateway* allows an incoming HTTP request and distributes it to the network based on the desired traffic rules. This makes it possible to communicate with the client application from any device to access the available games at any time, without the intervention of a third party, such as medical personnel.

Therefore, in COGNIPLAT platform each game is implemented as a separate microservice (see game-provider in Fig. 11). Each microservice contains the logic that describes which resources will be used for the game as well as whether an object needs to be created, and what its value will be according to the constraints specified in the ontology. Also, every service is accessible remotely through an API gateway. Figure 12 shows as an example the flow of messages that are exchanged between the COGNIPLAT platform microservices in order to create an instance of the game *Antonyms*.

All platform services accept requests in the JSON (JavaScript Object Notation) format and respond to the same formatting. Table 3 lists the supported endpoints of COGNILAT platform services where *{resource}* denotes one of the available games.

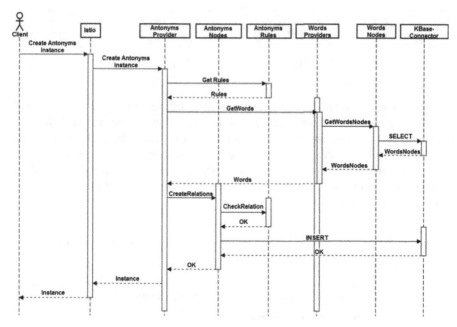

Fig. 12. Request flow for creating an instance of the game *Antonyms*.

Table 3. Endpoints of COGNILAT platform services [17].

HTTP verb	Resource URL	Response
GET	/mci/{resource}	All available game instances
POST	/mci/{resource}	A created game instance
GET	/mci/{resource}/{id}	A specific game instance
PUT	/mci/{resource}/{id}	Resolution of a specific game instance

3.5 Evaluation

To assess the perceived usability and technology acceptance of the COGNIPLAT platform an evaluation study was piloted with the participation of fifteen (15) healthy elderly with good average cognitive functionality (mean 68.7 ± 3.8 years, 6 female and 9 male). Several steps were undertaken by each participant during the evaluation process as shown in Fig. 13. After reading and signing the consent form, the Montreal Cognitive Assessment (MoCA) test [21] was completed by each participant to validate their cognitive functioning level. Then, a 45 min in-depth usage session of the game platform took place in the form of a rehabilitation simulation. Both qualitative and quantitative tools were used for assessing the game platform acceptance and usefulness in terms of completing the SUS (System Usability Scale) questionnaire [22] and conducting a semi-structured brief interview meeting.

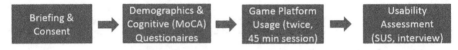

Fig. 13. Evaluation process steps.

The SUS questionnaire offers a reliable, valid and efficient tool to test system usability [23]. Furthermore, it is an effective tool, provided that it is concise including just 10 statements that can be applied to a broad variety of systems. The questionnaire items are affirmative and negative alternating statements rated on a five Likert scale from 1 (strongly disagree) to 5 (strongly agree). The wording of the original questionnaire items was adapted by replacing "system" with "game platform" to reflect the context of the study as shown in Table 4.

Table 4. SUS questionnaire items with affirmative and negative alternating statements.

ID	Statement
S1	I think that I would like to use this game platform frequently
S2	I found the game platform unnecessarily complex
S3	I thought the game platform was easy to use
S4	I think that I would need the support of a technical person to be able to use this game platform
S5	I found the various functions in this game platform were well integrated
S6	I thought there was too much inconsistency in this game platform
S7	I would imagine that most people would learn to use this game platform very quickly
S8	I found the game platform very cumbersome to use
S9	I felt very confident using the game platform
S10	I needed to learn a lot of things before I could get going with this game platform

The original scores of 0–40 for each participant were converted to 0–100 and the mean SUS score was found to be 80 (median = 85), indicating a high user acceptance [23]. Figure 14 outlines the SUS questionnaire results illustrating the distribution of the ratings for each statement. The participants have a strong perception that the usage of the game platform is characterized by simplicity, consistency and accessibility while the learning effort is acceptable as indicated by the responses in S2, S6, S8 and S10. Conversely, a more cautious feedback is provided regarding the ability of the participants to handle the game platform without external support. The latter is indicated by the responses in S4 and S9 which show that their intermediate ratings are stronger than the outer and more confident ratings. This observation is in accordance with other studies involving the usage and evaluation of technology-based solutions by the elderly emphasizing their variable familiarity with technology in addition to their general feeling of technology fear [24, 25].

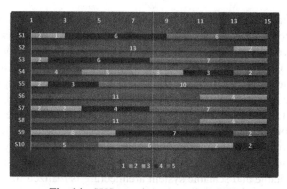

Fig. 14. SUS questionnaire ratings [17].

Qualitative data were also gathered by conducting a brief interview with each one participant. A semi-structured approach was followed and sample questions in the interview agenda included as follows:

- *Did you find the application easy to use?*
- *Were the games an easy and enjoyable way to practice your cognitive functions?*
- *Do you think that the time given to you in the games was sufficient, little or too much to complete?*
- *Which game did you like the most?*
- *Were there any of the games that you found unjustifiably difficult in your opinion? If so, which one?*

The analysis of the qualitative data collected confirms previous results showing that participants find the complexity of the system to be low, the interaction requirements of the game screens were easy to comprehend regarding their operations and the game mechanics didn't require much effort to use. A noteworthy comment made by several participants was that cognitive operations and in particular memory will probably improve gradually by training with the proposed exercises. Games that use multimedia resources were considered favorable with respect to text-based exercises by the majority of the participants. Such observations provide guidelines for improvements in future versions of the games.

4 Discussion

Healthcare applications in technology rich environments need to become more sustainable and effective. An approach to achieve this is to handle efficiently the knowledge and data that are characterizing the application domain. In this study we have examined different mental healthcare applications whose common characteristic is that they integrate ontology models in their operation, in order to organize the knowledge in the specific application domain of healthcare, developing systems that provide personalized services for the needs of each patient.

More specifically, the cognitive rehabilitation system, presented in Sect. 3, aims to show that an ontological approach allows the automatic creation of exercises for the rehabilitation of cognitive impaired older adults, offering on the one hand the possibility for each patient to exercise with new stimulus of multimedia resources, and on the other hand relieving the specialist from the work of producing these appropriate exercises, which until now were created by hand. The remote health monitoring and ontology-based architecture (Sect. 2.1) targets the development of a system that will be able to provide a good level of physical and mental health care, as well as seamless communication between the various heterogeneous entities involved in the system. By organizing the communication and data layer independently from the conceptual layer defined in the ontology, an adaptable and scalable system architecture is realized for supporting data exchange between different end points. The other two applications presented are more specific, as they aim at the care and treatment of patients suffering from dementia and suggest systems for the appropriate interventions, in case the patient is upset or confused. The augmented cognition system (Sect. 2.2) aims at the appropriate adaptation of the system operation, so that it can provide the best possible help to the patients, but also to their caregivers, while the confusion management system (Sect. 2.3) proposes methods of understanding the behavior of daily living conditions so that patients will be able to manage various ad hoc situations. A summary of the contribution and results of each application explored is presented in Table 5.

Table 5. Summary of ontology-based healthcare applications.

Application	Challenge	Approach	Ontology role	Ref
Remote health monitoring	Integrate heterogeneous components	Autonomic computing	Management and integration of homecare services	[9]
Interventions to address dementia related behaviors	Dealing with disturbing behaviors of people with dementia	Human-centered models of dementia care	Personalized intervention by selecting suitable services and adapting their operation according to the context	[11]
Home care for patients with Alzheimer	Monitoring and handling agitation behavior	Behavior understanding in everyday life	Reusable model for monitoring and managing confusion	[12]
Cognitive rehabilitation with SG	Addressing mild cognitive impairment in elderly	Game platform development	Automatic generation of cognitive training exercises	This work

In particular, this work has shown that an ontology-based approach is appropriate for the automatic generation of exercises for MCI rehabilitation purposes and the management of a wide range of (multimedia) stimuli. The outcome of our evaluation study shows that the cognitive level, the familiarity with the technology and the educational level are factors that affect the acceptability of the system. For the design of the games and their user interface we have followed a user-centered design approach from the beginning of the development process targeting a high usability and efficiency. According to the pilot evaluation that goal was achieved to a very good degree.

The broader goal of the COGNIPLAT platform is to make it easier for elderly with MCI to achieve an increased sense of self-efficacy by improving their functionality, which, according to recent research in neuropsychology, directly contributes to both cognitive and physical health. All of these play a crucial role in achieving our aim, as they allow seniors to apply the exercises for extended periods of time without getting tired. It is evident that more persistence in the exercises brings better recovery results.

Even though the importance of knowledge management via ontologies in healthcare applications has been demonstrated, there are still challenges and problems to overcome. Some of the challenges faced by ontology designers and developers are the following:

- In the healthcare domain there is a plethora of ontologies which makes it difficult to design a unified ontology that will include all the information contained in existing ontologies;
- The provision of different vocabularies for similar healthcare applications requires efficient strategies for ontology mapping and alignment to get common information into a comprehensible format;
- The lack of a standard or a methodology with appropriate criteria for tracking down a suitable ontology in a healthcare application domain, among a variety of similar ontologies, as well as the lack of a common methodology for reusing/analyzing existing ontologies;
- The lack of a unified update mechanism on the development of new ontologies in the healthcare field;
- The lack of commonly accepted standards for evaluating the quality of ontologies in the healthcare field;
- The lack of easy to use interfaces for browsing, querying and displaying the semantic healthcare information in a meaningful way;
- For the implementation of ontologies in languages such as OWL and RDF, some design standards have been proposed which, if followed, could facilitate the re-use or extension of ontologies, although they are not widely used;
- For developers without relevant background, the learning curve of OWL language and the required time to master the proper tools and technologies could be significant.

5 Conclusion and Future Work

In this paper, an ontology-based game platform for mild cognitive impairment rehabilitation was presented. The proposed approach emphasizes the development of personalized serious games for training cognitive skills by modelling both the static relationships of game resources and the dynamic game rules. From that standpoint it is possible to fuse the ontology knowledge with the associated dynamic knowledge reflected by these rules. Consequently, game tasks can be established through rules based on user preferences and conditions achieving thus personalization. The game platform operation is accessible from client applications through the HTTP protocol. In this way, the functionality can be accessed by any device (mobile, desktop etc.) and at any place (at care center, at home etc.).

As a future work, the stored data from the game usage can be processed by machine learning algorithms to determine more effective exercise plans to improve the required cognitive skills, whereas the discovery of patterns can assist the classification of patients to diagnostic levels. This functionality is expected that will increase more the engagement of the users and their willingness for continuous practicing with the platform.

Even though the importance of semantic web technologies in healthcare field is broadly accepted, there are still challenges and problems to overcome. One such challenge is that knowledge engineering and representing special-purpose activities such as the game mechanics for cognitive rehabilitation to ontology hierarchies are challenging and demanding tasks. Ontology maintenance (e.g. the extension of the game platform with new games) is another challenge. Developing tools to automate these tasks are essential. Likewise the development of effective interfaces leveraging on new architectural styles such as microservices to build and deploy rapidly proof-of-concept applications will increase the assertiveness on ontology usefulness in the healthcare domain. Finally, machine learning techniques can be applied for extracting new knowledge, however issues, such as administering data quality are preconditions for obtaining valuable insights.

Acknowledgements. This research has been co-financed by the European Regional Development Fund of the European Union and Greek national funds through the Operational Program Competitiveness, Entrepreneurship and Innovation, under the call ERA-NETS 2018 (ID:T8EPA2-00011, grant MIS:5041669). The authors would like to thank the fellow researchers in the COGNIPLAT project for their valuable support in the performed research and the volunteers that took part in the evaluation study.

References

1. Weber-Jahnke, J., Peyton, L., Topaloglou, T.: eHealth system interoperability. Inf. Syst. Front. **14**(1), 1–3 (2012)
2. Cannoy, S.D., Iyer, L.: Semantic Web standards and ontologies in the medical sciences and healthcare. In: Semantic Web Technologies and E-Business: Toward the Integrated Virtual Organization and Business Process Automation, pp. 405–420. IGI Global (2007)
3. Corcho, O., Fernández-López, M., Gómez-Pérez, A.: Ontological engineering: principles, methods, tools and languages. In: Calero C., Ruiz F., Piattini M. (eds) Ontologies for Software Engineering and Software Technology, pp. 1–48. Springer, Heidelberg (2006). https://doi.org/10.1007/3-540-34518-3_1
4. Cardillo, E., Eccher, C., Serafini, L., Tamilin, A.: Logical analysis of mappings between medical classification systems. In: Dochev, D., Pistore, M., Traverso, P. (eds.) AIMSA 2008. LNCS (LNAI), vol. 5253, pp. 311–321. Springer, Heidelberg (2008). https://doi.org/10.1007/978-3-540-85776-1_26

5. McBride, B. (2004). The resource description framework (RDF) and its vocabulary description language RDFS. In: Staab, S., Studer, R. (eds.) Handbook on Ontologies, pp. 51–65. Springer, Heidelberg. https://doi.org/10.1007/978-3-540-24750-0_3

6. Welty, C., McGuinness, D.L., Smith, M.K.: Owl web ontology language guide. W3C recommendation, W3C (2004). https://www.w3.org/TR/2004/REC-owl-guide-20040210/

7. Paganelli, F., Giuli, D.: An ontology-based system for context-aware and configurable services to support home-based continuous care. IEEE Trans. Inf Technol. Biomed. **15**(2), 324–333 (2010)

8. Skillen, K.L., Chen, L., Nugent, C.D., Donnelly, M.P., Burns, W., Solheim, I.: Ontological user modelling and semantic rule-based reasoning for personalisation of Help-On-Demand services in pervasive environments. Future Gener. Comput. Syst. **34**, 97–109 (2014)

9. Lasierra, N., Alesanco, A., Garcia, J.: Designing an architecture for monitoring patients at home: ontologies and web services for clinical and technical management integration. IEEE J. Biomed. Health Inform. **18**(3), 896–906 (2013)

10. Lasierra, N., Alesanco, A., Guillén, S., García, J.: A three stage ontology-driven solution to provide personalized care to chronic patients at home. J. Biomed. Inform. **46**(3), 516–529 (2013)

11. Navarro, R.F., Rodríguez, M.D., Favela, J.: Intervention tailoring in augmented cognition systems for elders with dementia. IEEE J. Biomed. Health Inform. **18**(1), 361–367 (2013)

12. Fook, V.F.S., Tay, S.C., Jayachandran, M., Biswas, J., Zhang, D.: An ontology-based context model in monitoring and handling agitation behavior for persons with dementia. In: Fourth Annual IEEE International Conference on Pervasive Computing and Communications Workshops (PERCOMW 2006), p. 5. IEEE, March 2006

13. Brickley, D., Miller, L.: FOAF vocabulary specification 0.91 (2007)

14. Arnab, S., Dunwell, I., Debattista, K.: Serious Games for Healthcare: Applications and Implications. Medical Information Science Reference (2013)

15. Gauthier, S., et al.: Mild cognitive impairment. Lancet **367**(9518), 1262–1270 (2006)

16. Brandão, J., Cunha, P., Carvalho, V.H., Soares, F.O.: An overview of serious games in cognitive rehabilitation. In: Encyclopedia of E-Health and Telemedicine, pp. 744–753. IGI Global (2016)

17. Goumopoulos, C., Igoumenakis, I.: An ontology based game platform for mild cognitive impairment rehabilitation. In: ICT4AWE, pp. 130–141 (2020)

18. Gerling, K.M., Schulte, F.P., Smeddinck, J., Masuch, M.: Game design for older adults: effects of age-related changes on structural elements of digital games. In: International Conference on Entertainment Computing, pp. 235–242 (2012)

19. Bechhofer, S., et al.: OWL web ontology language reference. W3C Recommendation, vol. 10, no. 02 (2004)

20. Motik, B., et al.: OWL 2 web ontology language: structural specification and functional-style syntax. W3C Recommendation, vol. 27, no. 65, p. 159 (2009)

21. Nasreddine, Z.S., et al.: The montreal cognitive assessment, MoCA: a brief screening tool for mild cognitive impairment. J. Am. Geriatr. Soc. **53**(4), 695–699 (2005)

22. Brooke, J.: SUS-A quick and dirty usability scale. Usability Eval. Ind. **189**(194), 4–7 (1996)

23. Bangor, A., Kortum, P.T., Miller, J.T.: An empirical evaluation of the system usability scale. Int. J. Hum.-Comput. Interact. **24**(6), 574–594 (2008)

24. Goumopoulos, C., Papa, I., Stavrianos, A.: Development and evaluation of a mobile application suite for enhancing the social inclusion and well-being of seniors. In: Informatics, vol. 4, no. 3, p. 15, September 2017

25. Chartomatsidis, M., Goumopoulos, C.: A balance training game tool for seniors using microsoft kinect and 3D worlds. In: International Conference on Information and Communication Technologies for Ageing Well and e-Health, pp. 135–145 (2019)

26. Newman, S.: Building Microservices: Designing Fine-Grained Systems. O'Reilly Media, Inc. (2015)
27. Prasanna, D.R.: Dependency Injection. Manning Publications, Shelter Island (2009)

Author Index

Printed in the United States
By Bookmasters